# Shape Up!

Progressive Fitness For Practical People

## Vic Sanders

*to every person
who is interested
not in getting more
years out of their life
but rather in
GETTING MORE LIFE OUT OF THEIR YEARS*

McGraw-Hill Ryerson Limited
Toronto   Montreal   New York   London

**Shape Up!**

Progressive Fitness For Practical People

ISBN 0-07-082292-1

1 2 3 4 5 6 7 8 9 10 D 4 3 2 1 0 9 8 7 6 5

Printed and bound in Canada

# Acknowledgements

Ontario Government Ministry of Tourism for their co-operation in helping me select pictures of fit people participating in various sporting activities.

The Adidas (Canada) Company Limited who supplied all our outfits.

My friend and associate Doug Miller who practically stood on his head to take pictures at the various angles I felt necessary.

Two great people who put up with me day after day and then volunteered their time and efforts during the taking of all the exercise pictures: Wendy Cecil-Stewart and Jim Henderson.

Also, thanks to John Gibson, Barney Bayliss, Melanie Bright, Wendy Cecil-Stewart, and Jim Henderson for the cover photo.

# Preface

Today, as never before, governments and private enterprise are spending more and more to promote fitness: fitness through sports, fitness through exercise —in general, fitness through more activity.

One of the underlying reasons for this general concern is the cost of providing health and sickness insurance and the overwhelming loss of productivity through lost working hours due largely to avoidable illness. We are told that doing something is better than doing nothing. No one would argue with such a statement, but it is even better to be doing enough of the right kind of things, and have those things in turn do us some good.

In this book I have made suggestions on what to do, how to do it, how often it should be done, and some suggestions about where it should be done. We are striving for basic conditioning of the body rather than frustrating the mind; therefore, I do not recommend exercise studios, health spas, commercial gymnasiums, or massage and body rub parlors where the instruction is given by vivacious, topless young ladies. These institutions may or may not have their place, but all you are likely to get is an overtaxed body, confused explanations of what you are doing and why, and probably an empty pocket-book for your trouble. I do not advocate the quick, easy methods of getting your body into condition. Don't be fooled into thinking that mechanical devices that do all the work while the body just jiggles along will put you in condition. Aside from their general uselessness, such devices can lead to minor and possibly serious complications. However, many mechanical and semi-mechanical aids that force the body to exercise can be very useful; I have not discussed these in any detail, however, since I believe it is better to condition the body using the body as your guide to how far you can or should develop. I have discussed diet and also why I believe the normal healthy person who exercises properly and regularly and eats nourishing foods should have no reason to diet.

I don't presume to have all the answers. I sometimes wonder if I have enough. However, I do believe, through my own experiences and the experiences of those people who regularly join in my program, that diets, crash exercise programs, mechanical devices, etc. are not necessary in order to stay slim, trim and alive. Best of all, this program *won't cost you a cent.*

Vic Sanders

# Contents

# You want to Feel Young and Alive

You're overweight or underweight. You've tried this diet, that diet, done this, done that, bought this or that cream for your face, bought this lotion for your body, stopped drinking (but only temporarily), stopped eating for a while, cut out fats, starches, etc.—it goes on and on and for what? Ninety-nine per cent of it turns out to be a flop in the end because you are searching for an easy way out of a rather uneasy situation. In our desire to be slim, trim and look like the gorgeous creatures we see in the ads in magazines, in movies or on television we try one thing after the other.

Why do we do this? We do it so we will appear younger than we are and more desirable than we probably are. Tucked away in our subconscious is that false belief that if we appear younger than we are we may live longer.

How can you or I or anyone else possibly tell if anybody lived a day longer because he exercised or didn't? We don't know.

Many studies have been done on the benefits of exercising to overall body functioning. It has been proven over and over again that physically fit people are far less prone to catch many common diseases, for example, the common cold. There is no proof or guarantee, however, that you won't.

Studies have proven that through a good fitness program you can and usually do reduce your heart beats per minute. If you make your heart work less but more efficiently, it's possible that it might last longer. Again it hasn't been proven that you live longer, but while you are living you are not putting your vital organs under as great a strain.

The heart after all is a muscle, undoubtedly the most important muscle we have. Like all muscles it must be used and strengthened. If not, when it is called upon in time of stress or strain (to shovel snow, push a stalled car, climb extra stairs, etc.) it cramps up like any other muscle, ceases to function, at best temporarily, and we have a heart attack. It could happen to a fit person but the probability is much less, and if it does the possibility of recovery is much greater. Studies have also shown that most people in our society don't necessarily grow old or wear out, but rather "rust" out.

This seems reason enough to exercise. However, I have my own philosophy of why I exercise and want to: it's not that I want more years out of my life, it's simply that I want more LIFE out of my years. If I do live longer because I've stayed healthy—and I think that's a good assumption—then the extra years are an added bonus.

# Get Hooked on a New Routine

I know so many people at forty (and some who are younger) who can't wait to get home from a hard day at work, have a drink or two, have a snack (more often than not "junk food"), have a quick un-nutritious dinner and collapse in front of the television. They bring along a package of cigarettes and, of course, a few beers or a bottle just to make the evening a little more enjoyable. What a dull existence.

Is it so necessary to rush home from work to this routine? Think about it. Do we really need food at that hour, right after work? It's just habit and probably not a healthy one at that, because we are probably still so uptight from work and the ride home in traffic that the most we can hope to get out of the evening meal is a good case of indigestion. Why not go home or to the club, change into your gym clothes and get hooked on a new routine. Go for a run or a workout and get rid of your day's frustrations and aggressions.

Better still, enlist a friend, neighbour or fellow worker who is in the same rut to join in with you. There are times when you'll need the moral support and companionship. When you have finally eaten, it is wise to let your food digest for an hour before you take on any strenuous exercise or chores, but don't be fooled by the theory that you shouldn't do anything after a meal. I often take a leisurely swim or walk after dinner. There's really nothing better. It helps the digestive system and you feel better besides. Don't misunderstand me, however; I do not suggest that you go on a marathon swim or walk; that is strenuous exercise and it shouldn't be done for at least an hour after eating.

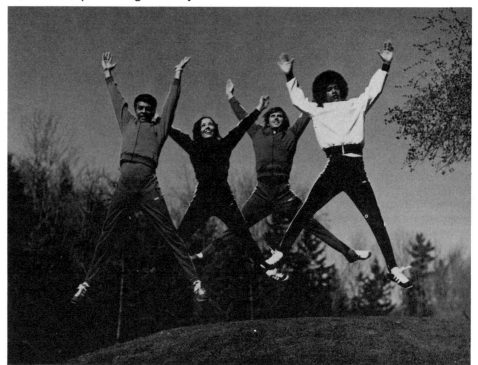

# Why Should I Exercise

How, you say, can all that exercise be good for me when I'm tense and have so many problems from work weighing on my mind. Amazing, isn't it, how we all seem to have all the problems and the other guy doesn't have any.

Believe it or not, I go to work at a regular nine-to-five type job. I think I have to face as many problems and frustrations as anybody else. What do workouts do for me? They let me take out all my frustrations on the track or the gym floor; I am able to clear away all the cobwebs and then my problems seem to become smaller and the solutions to those problems become easier.

We all want to live more active lives and a lot of us, I believe, try to learn the secrets of perpetual health. Well, there is no secret solution and I don't believe there is such a thing as perpetual health. But exercise, good physical exercise, will go a long way to giving a more active life and far better health.

So now you're convinced you want to live a more active life, but you like sports better than exercising. Don't confuse exercise with sport. Exercise is not a sport, it is a program that should enable you to par-ticipate in the sports of your choice with more vigor and vitality. It will allow you to enjoy participating in sports to a much greater degree.

Or it may be a conditioning program can enable you to get the gardening done, repairs made, paint the room you've been promising to do for the last six months, and a hundred and one other things that you've always wanted to do, but never had the initiative or energy for. You will also do these things with a greater sense of satisfaction. In short, a good exercise program enables you to condition yourself to live and get more out of life.

The basic program I have outlined takes about half an hour. I can just hear the cries going up: "I can't spare a half hour!" Well, *you* know and *I* know that busy people think in terms of productivity. Business watch-words are: volume, output, return on investment, and of course dollars and cents, to name just a few. The tempo is fast, many times frantic. Things must be done now, tomorrow, or often yesterday. We drive ourselves in business and we drive the people we work with. All this means long hours, strain, and a consumption of nervous energy with altogether too little time spent considering our bodies' demands for health and fitness.

We carefully maintain the business equipment we own or have re-sponsibility for as well as the enter-prises we run and the men and women who make them operate, but so often shamefully neglect the most important piece of equipment —ourselves.

It doesn't matter whether you are a lawyer, manufacturer, stockbroker, insurance salesman, store clerk, la-borer, supervisor, foreman or com-pany president—whether you cre-ate or direct, supervise or follow— you have an obligation to yourself and your job to maintain peak per-formance in your body and mind, as you have to maintain peak per-formance in business and industry. Without a good exercise program, such as the one suggested in this book, the body cannot be expected to function at its optimum level.

# What is Physical Fitness

I suppose physical fitness means a lot of different things to different people. In many clinical studies, for example, fitness is related to the functioning of the heart, blood vessels, respiratory system, muscular system, and so forth.

An athletic coach, on the other hand, may think of fitness in terms of the level of conditioning for a particular sport. The fitness training of world champion sprinters differs a great deal from the fitness training for an olympic hockey team, and, by the same token, the kind of physical preparation for professional football players will not resemble that of competitive swimmers.

The mid-week athlete out for a game with the guys or gals, or the weekend golfer should be able to enjoy the total game or activity, not only half of it. This type of person needs general body conditioning and muscle toning.

The person who does not participate in any given sport also needs a general conditioning program, for it is in this category above all that most problems occur when the body is called upon to perform a little extra. Throughout all these various approaches to physical fitness, however, there is a common concern for one thing—output.

We can describe physical fitness as being the ability to undertake daily physical tasks and engage in a favorite activity without undue fatigue. Obviously fitness will be the major factor in the interest, enthusiasm, enjoyment, and success that you can expect to experience in your personal efforts, be they physical or mental.

It is most important to point out that the conditioning or exercise program is not and *should not* be considered an end in itself. A conditioning program is a method by which we prepare the body for the sports or other activities in which we wish to participate.

The general conditioning program I have outlined in this book is an overall plan suited equally well for the amateur or professional athlete, business man, labourer, housewife, secretary, stockbroker, and *you*. It is not geared to any given sport, but is related through the variety of exercises shown to a wide variety of recreational and competitive activities. Above all it is a practical approach to conditioning the body for a happier, healthier life.

# How, How Much, How Often

Fitness can only be obtained through regular physical activity. The kind and intensity of activity and the amount of time you devote to it will determine in large part the level of conditioning you can expect to attain.

One of the keys to any successful program of conditioning is the progression from lighter intensity to more strenuous workouts. Your body will adjust without too many complaints if you gradually increase the demands you make upon it. Also, the amount of time to be spent on physical activity over an extended period of time is difficult to state without knowing the individual's specific goals. To attain a reasonable level of fitness for the average man or woman, a half hour daily appears to be sufficient. To maintain this level of fitness once it is attained, a half hour regularly three times per week on alternate days will probably do the trick. This, of course, would be totally unsatisfactory to the professional athlete. Think of your physical fitness in terms of levels on a personal scale. By seeking to maintain a level of general physical fitness throughout the year, you will be able to raise your fitness level steadily, efficiently and economically to the peak required for satisfactory achievement. Don't be discouraged by the aches and pains and stiffness that you are going to encounter during the first few workouts. Such aches and pains are simply nature's way of telling you that in the past you haven't been doing your physical homework and it's now time to pay. When the aches and pains rear their ugly head, simply go back to your program and work them out. If you give in by saying, "But I can't today, I ache too much," and you nurse the aches and pains during the initial stages, the next time you exercise you will encounter the same problems all over again.

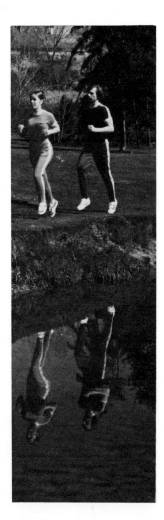

# Who Should Exercise

Every normal healthy person, regardless of superficial differences and a thousand excuses, should face the truth of the matter that if we exercised regularly and properly many of our problems probably would not exist.

Remember the poor old woman who went to the doctor, and, when he told her she really had nothing wrong with her, said, "How dare you tell me there's nothing wrong with me! Whatever will I tell my friends?" A lot of people say to me, "Oh, if I were younger, I would probably get into an exercise program, but I'm too old for that now." I usually say to them, "How old will you be in five years time if you don't exercise, and how old will you be in five years time if you do?" The answer is just the same; therefore, the best time to start exercising is now.

We all have had our ups and downs, some minor, some major, but if we have had the good fortune to come through it all in reasonably good shape, we should start on our personal rebuilding program now. Don't let the past take an unnecessary toll on the future.

If you are much over forty and have not lived an active life, or if you are in some way handicapped, or have had a heart attack or some other serious illness, consult your doctor before you start. If necessary, set up a program with your doctor and a physical education counsellor. Then watch yourself become your own miracle worker.

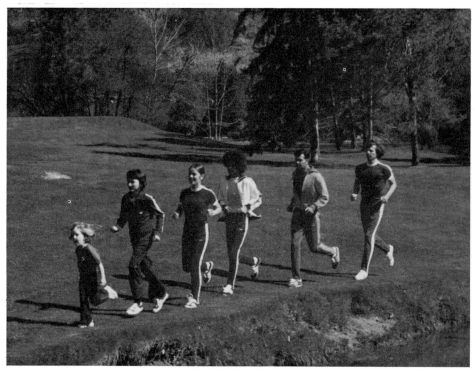

# Where to Get Started

Having decided to embark on an exercise program, the most important question seems to be, "Where should I go?" Check your basement or bedroom. Usually you will find that the basement offers excellent usable space with good ventilation and a degree of privacy to boot. A large amount of space is not that important. All you need is sufficient room to swing your arms in a full circle upwards and sideways.

If you feel a little company would be advantageous, recruit your family, neighbours or friends. If you have the facilities you can enjoy backyard group sessions, still allowing each of you to follow your own program.

We often find that doing things in a group atmosphere helps each individual: others striving for similar goals often gives us that little extra drive, something so important to an exercise program.

Apartment buildings offer another good source of space. There are usually recreation rooms or rooms set aside for tenant activities. A group of tenants that wishes to form an exercise group will usually find the superintendant most helpful.

If you prefer a more formal program, you can choose any of a number of places. Let me give you a few suggestions, but don't consider these the only places worthy of mention. Try your local "Y", check with your local board of education, community college, university or recognized fitness institute.

The program offered will probably vary as much as the name of the organization, so I suggest you find out if their program is designed to satisfy your particular needs. If it is a formal program, compare it to the type outlined in this book. If you don't feel any of these programs fit your needs, set up your own program or organize your own group by recruiting your friends or business associates. If you are in a formal group already it will undoubtedly help if you concentrate on the more difficult exercises at home following the descriptions outlined in this book. I cannot overemphasize that self-motivation is the prime ingredient; we must want to feel better to look better and be more satisfied with our accomplishments. The group environment encourages us to exercise more regularly because it shows us that no one can achieve perfection or do everything at once. It is human nature that we try to avoid those exercises that demand the most exertion, but unfortunately we usually need those exercises most.

The physical fitness and conditioning program you become involved in should provide these ingredients:

1. Regular relaxation by relieving many of your frustrations and tensions.
2. Physical exertion that will improve your cardiovascular (heart) and respiratory (breathing) systems.
3. Toning the various muscle groups in the body without necessarily building excess muscle tissue.
4. Improvement of your flexibility, agility, balance, and endurance.

This type of productive physical exercise will lead you to a healthier body and a more alert mind.

# You and Your Diet

I often feel it is unfortunate that we live in a diet-conscious era. The continual stream of conflicting information constantly thrown at us from all sides about what we should and should not eat can probably do us more harm than good. I say to every normal healthy person, "Forget the diets!" The end result of allowing our weight to fluctuate up and down is often unhealthy and disastrous to most of us anyway.

Snacks are not the answer, nor is junk food, but meat, fish, potatoes, and vegetables most certainly are. Search out the casserole dishes or the multitude of other one-dish meals that most cookbooks today offer; they taste great and take little preparation. Most of them can be prepared ahead of time, so that they can be popped into the oven without bother when you arrive home from work or workout.

With a good exercise program we shouldn't need a special diet as we will consume sufficient calories to offset the calorie outflow. What we consume, however, with the proper calorie balance is important.

The proper exercise program will enable you to lose weight if you are overweight and the reverse will tend to take place if you are underweight. Proper exercise will also cause your weight to redistribute if necessary so that it is where it should be and not where it shouldn't be.

# Can You Relax

I believe that one of our greatest joys of life is being able to truly relax. And yet during our hectic everyday life we seldom if ever take time to just relax. We work through lunch or go out for lunch with a client to talk business or with some of our fellow workers to discuss problems. Lunch should be a time to relax, to talk about non-business activities, that trip you are planning, that special project you have undertaken at home, your favourite hobby, but certainly not about work. The mid-morning or mid-afternoon coffee break has long lost its original intent. It has turned into a cup of coffee at a meeting rather than a time to relax.

We come home in the evening with a stuffed brief-case full of the day's problems. I suppose we think we can relax at home and solve the problems. If you're like I used to be, you probably stare at it, too tired to open it, and feel guilty all evening because you haven't opened it. I discovered a long time ago that if we want to accomplish more in our daily life, we must learn to relax. Take a short ten to fifteen minute break mid-way through the morning and afternoon, but make it a complete break. Shut your office door and lie down on the couch, if you should be lucky enough to have one.

If you don't have an office where you can shut the door, leave your work area and go to the coffee shop or lounge, shut your eyes and let your mind wander for the ten to fifteen minutes.

This exercise will relax you; do eight or ten wide arm rotations and take eight or ten good deep breaths. Let your head and neck go limp and heavy and your sholders sag for a few seconds. It will do wonders for you. A good exercise program of course provides another time of great relaxation. After your workout, a good hot lingering shower, steam bath or sauna is the perfect relaxant. You will feel the body tingle and the weight of the day's problems seem to wash away. Learn to relax at your sports activities. Try to work out tensions and nervous compulsions. Remember, top notch athletes remain *cool* under pressure. Participate in the sports of your choice as often as you can to simply enjoy them. We all strive to do better, but don't let the desire for perfection interfere with the sheer enjoyment of participating in the sports you have chosen. The frustrated golfer who smashes an iron over the nearest fencepost or throws a club into the stream isn't enjoying a relaxing game of golf.

So often I hear people say, "I'll go home, have a few drinks and relax." How wrong they are; alcohol is not a relaxant—it is a *depressant*! I enjoy a drink to be social, but not to help me relax.

# The Exercise Program

Today as never before we are being bombarded with all sorts of theories on "Instant Fitness," "Total Fitness in Thirty Minutes a Week," "Five Exercises to Perfect Fitness," etc., etc. Who are they kidding? There's no such thing as instant fitness and 30 minutes per week is a waste of time. There are no five single exercises that will produce overall physical fitness, at least not to my knowledge and in my experience.

Professor Thomas Kirk Cureton, Ph.D., of the University of Illinois, who is one of the world's leading fitness authorities, says, "It may be the hardest work you ever do. But it may also save your life . . ."

Dr. Cureton demands and, from those who work with him, gets 60 minutes of vigorous activity each day. Scornfully, he rejects all forms of "instant fitness". "You tell the public the wrong thing and they spend their time doing the inadequate. That keeps them from getting fit," he says. "If you tell them the right thing to do, then they have some chance."

Like Dr. Cureton, I believe that too often we are told to do something in the name of fitness that is wrong and that in fact will not help us to get fit.

I have a friend who claims to be a fitness nut. He sure is—he set up a gym in his basement. Hurrah, said I, another convert to the healthy life. Maybe he'll abandon all the diets, instant body-beautiful gimmicks, etc. You know what he did? Went out and spent quite a few hundred dollars on fancy equipment to make him the picture of health overnight. He wound up with bruises and a very sore back. Finally he came to me and said, "Vic, how do I go about getting into your program? I've got to do something."

My approach is simple, straightforward, and requires no special equipment. Your desire to shape up your body is all you need.

In any conditioning program you must place considerable emphasis on cardiovascular and respiratory improvement to build stamina. You must let yourself freely perspire. So often we hear that it is not lady-like or gentlemanly to sweat. Let's not kid ourselves; if we stop perspiring we are in trouble. Perspiration is simply our body's way of controlling temperature.

To achieve a reasonable level of overall fitness, even the beginner must exercise at least one half hour in effective length. The advanced programs often run as long as three quarters of an hour and specialty programs usually run for a full hour. The exercises for all levels are basically the same; only the intensity varies. For the specialty programs, after the basic conditioning program, special emphasis is placed on those parts of the body that will demand extra stress and strain when participating in specific sports.

The basic format should be followed in almost any general conditioning program, whether for an individual or a group. We begin by warming up the body to a point where perspiration is running freely and the pulse is substantilly increased. This usually takes from 5 to 7 minutes.

The warm-up is followed by the loosen-up. These are the short bending and easy stretching exercises used mainly in a preparatory way for the next phase of the program which consists of deep bending and stretching.

At the conclusion of the deep bending and stretching portion of the program, we usually have another short run to ensure that the body is properly reheated prior to the muscle toning portion of our program.

The muscle toning section of our program is basically the endurance and strength segment. This part of the program, is not, however, a muscle *building* program. Any muscle building that results suffices to bring the muscle density up to its required level. It is usual for a person with a large frame to carry a greater degree of muscle and flesh than a small framed person.

The muscle toning exercises range from the upper body (shoulders, chest, neck, upper back and upper arms), continuing down to the upper and middle abdomen, then moving to the lower abdomen, thighs, groin, and legs.

The program ends with one of the more important aspects of any exercise program, that being a cooldown and relaxation period. It is important that after any strenuous program you do not come to an abrupt conclusion. Return the body to its normal pulse rate and body temperature gradually.

# Exercising to Music

One of the things that can make exercising more enjoyable is to use music. In my sessions I have set each phase of the program to music.

To do this it is most important to plan the program first. Determine what you want to do and how long you wish to concentrate on each phase of your own program. I have made suggestions on how long you should spend on each phase. However, your particular needs may dictate that you should place a greater concentration in certain areas, thereby changing the length of your program.

Once you have designed your program select music that you can exercise to. The music should contain the correct beat or count to go along with the exercises being performed. For example, when you are running the beat should be steady and fast enough to give you a beat each time one of your feet touch the ground. In the loosen-up section of the program the beat should be a two count rhythm as it should for the push-up portion of the muscle toning. For the deep bending segment of your workout and the middle body section of the muscle toning the count must be four.

Do not try to exercise to just any music. If you wish to use just background music, you may select almost any type of music but it should be played very softly so it will not confuse the program.

# Preparing Your Own Program

## HELPFUL HINTS

Every good program requires a plan to be successful, not a hodge-podge of bends and grinds. Remember, there is no one best program for developing physical fitness, but some basic rules should be followed.

## Performing the Exercises

For the individual, you are your own leader. For the group leader, you must consider the needs of the group.

Plan your program ahead of time and develop a general outline of it. Review your program as you progress and be ready to make any required changes. Stress weak points and be flexible.

Make the program a challenge and a part of each person's life. For the individual, you will not wish to slacken off. Also, a challenge ensures good group attendance and progress.

For the group leader, become a part of the group, not an observer. Let the group see you striving also.

Arrive at the class early and meet new people; learn about them and their desires. Give them special instructions as necessary on starting out on their program.

Set a good pace for yourself, one that will make you work. For the group leader, remember that the pace you set must suit the majority of the class and not only do those exercises you find easy. Gear your program to the average ability of your group.

Be encouraging. Never openly criticize. A good sense of humor is a necessity for the group leader as well as the individual. Don't be afraid to laugh at yourself, but *not* at others.

In the group environment project your voice. Let everyone know exactly what you are going to do next. The body should move at a rhythmic pace and it is much better to make the movements slow and deliberate than jerky and unco-ordinated.

## The Planned Program

The key to a successful program lies in the sequence of exercises. Remember: Warm-Up; Loosen-Up; Stretching, Bending, and Pulling; Muscle Toning; and Cool-Down.

Make sure your program flows smoothly from exercise to exercise and phase to phase.

After the beginner phase of your program, rest periods should come only in the form of lighter, low intensity exercises.

Be sure your program includes exercises for each muscle group. Don't avoid those exercises that you find most difficult to execute. Those are the ones you need most!

## Participation

Participation is the key to the success of your program, whether it is you the individual or you the group leader.

Encourage the participants to attend by gearing the class to their ability.

As the group leader you must participate and identify with the group.

Discuss the program with your group: solicit suggestions and listen to them. I get very good ideas from my classes and they appreciate that I listen and act on useful suggestions.

## Your Program Format

The program has three levels. Be sure that you set your program to the correct level, for a program too easy will discourage you and your class as quickly as a program too hard.

*The Beginner Level* is for the person totally out of condition. These people have not participated in sports activities or other exercise for some time.

*The Intermediate Level* is for the person who has progressed through the beginner level or has been active in other forms of exercise or sport.

*The Advanced Level* is for the person who has progressed through the intermediate level or has a good recent record in strenuous sports like football, hockey, swimming, and water skiing.

Remember that the format at all levels is virtually the same; only the intensity and duration vary.

## WEAR APPROPRIATE CLOTHES

What you wear is so important. The wrong clothes can not only interfere with your exercising, but also certain fabrics can be hazardous to your well-being.

For outdoor jogging in the winter wear a sweat suit that will absorb the perspiration, yet protect you from the elements.

For outdoor jogging in the summer or in the summer rain, a T-shirt and shorts are the best. Some manufacturers have a good nylon jogging suit for summer rain, but it is not as comfortable as shorts and a T-shirt.

Avoid form-fitting garments which restrict freedom of movement. Remember that you are exercising, not putting on a fashion show.

Avoid plastic or rubberized garments which do not "breathe". You prespire to maintain an even body temperature; these garments do not absorb perspiration, causing harmful temperature build-up.

Get good shoes. Shoes should have a good arch support, be flexible, and have good gripping rubber soles.

Good sweat socks are important, because they add an additional cushion to your feet and absorb perspiration. They also help to prevent foot blisters.

For the men a good athletic supporter is essential.

For women a sports brassiere and long-line cotton underpants are advisable for comfort and support.

# The Warm-Up

The warm-up is designed specifically to prepare the body for the exercise program.

Upon completion of the warm-up phase you should be moderately perspiring, you should have an increased heart beat and your body should be sufficiently loose to prevent pulled muscles or other such injuries.

The warm-up period should be completed at a moderate pace.

The warm-up period may be extended to include any of the additional activities shown, but must include those exercises designated with an asterisk.

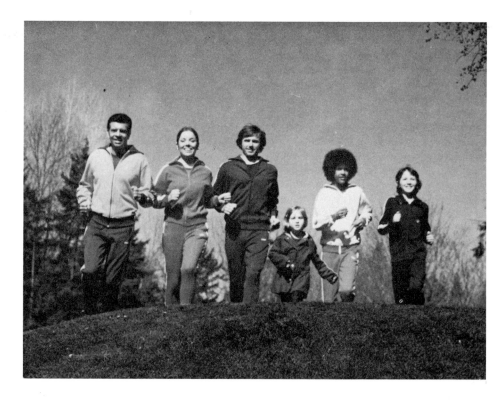

# EXERCISE 1  RUNNING ON THE SPOT*

(Note: Exercise 2 is an alternate to
          Exercise 1)

## Starting Position

Stand erect, feet 8 to 10 inches
apart.

## Action

Imitate running by bringing knees
up high at a rather rapid pace.

## Duration

Beginners      : 1 minute
Intermediate : 2 minutes
Advanced      : 3 minutes

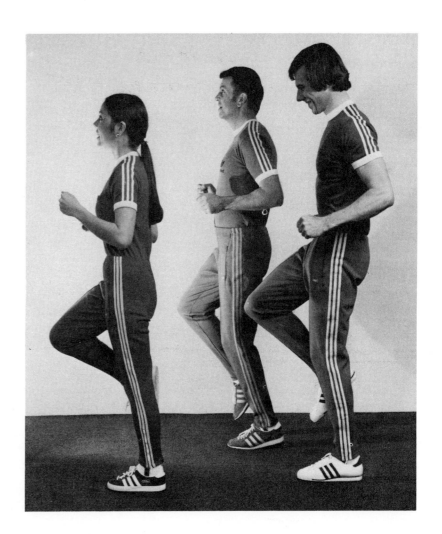

## EXERCISE 2   JOGGING*

### Starting Position

Stand erect but lean slightly forward. Let the body propel itself forward.

### Action

Raise left leg until left heel is about at level of right calf. Kick forward until right heel leaves ground. As you lower left leg push off on ball of right foot.
*Note:* When jogging land on ball of foot and lower your heel.

### Duration

Beginners     : 1 minute
Intermediate : 2 minutes
Advanced     : 3 minutes

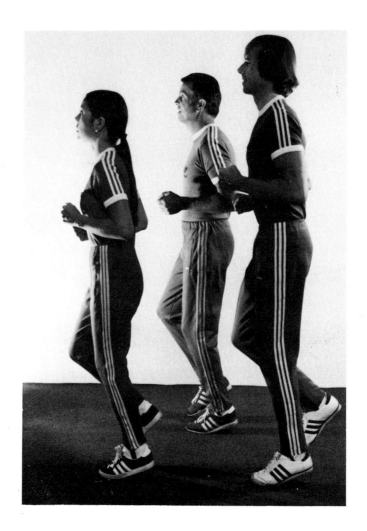

## EXERCISE 3   RUNNING*

### Starting Position

Stand erect but lean slightly forward. Let the body propel itself forward.

### Action

As in jogging, step out with left leg but stretch out further, propelling the body forward at a faster pace.

### Duration

Beginners    : ¼ mile
Intermediate : ¼ mile
Advanced     : ¼ – ½ mile

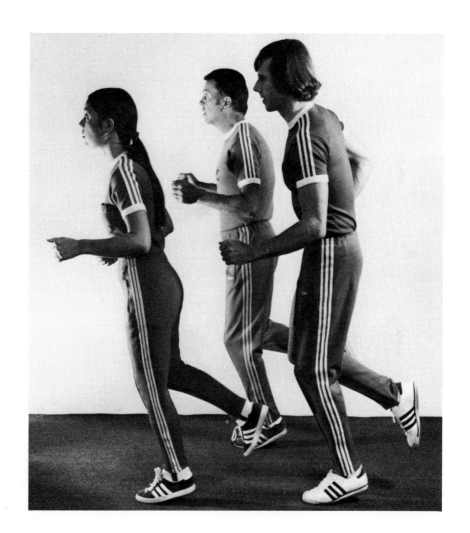

## EXERCISE 4   SPRINTING

### Starting Position

When sprinting you must first be jogging. When you reach end of gym, track etc., turn.

### Action

Lean well forward, arms bent. Push down with ball of foot thrusting opposite leg out as fast as possible. Dash to opposite end of sprint area. Jog to opposite end of sprint area and repeat.

### Duration

Beginners     : Sprint one length, jog one length: repeat 2 times.
Intermediate : Sprint one length, jog one length: repeat 4 times.
Advanced      : Sprint 2 or 3 lengths, jog one length: repeat 3 or 4 times.

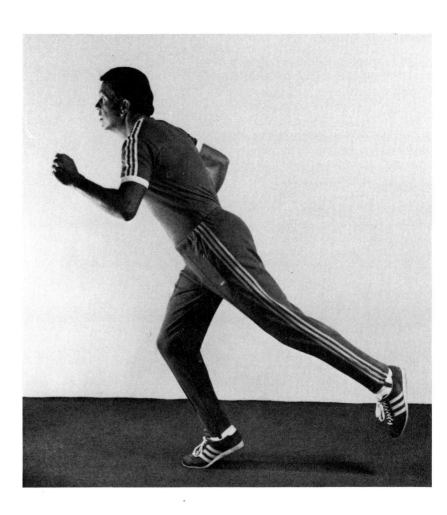

## EXERCISE 5   ARM CIRCLES

### Starting Position

Walking erect, shoulders back, arms extended to the sides at shoulder height, palms up.

### Action

Move arms in small circles in a backwards motion. With palms turned down, move arms in a forward motion.

### Repetitions

Beginners    : 8 times each way
Intermediate : 8 times each way
Advanced     : 8 times each way

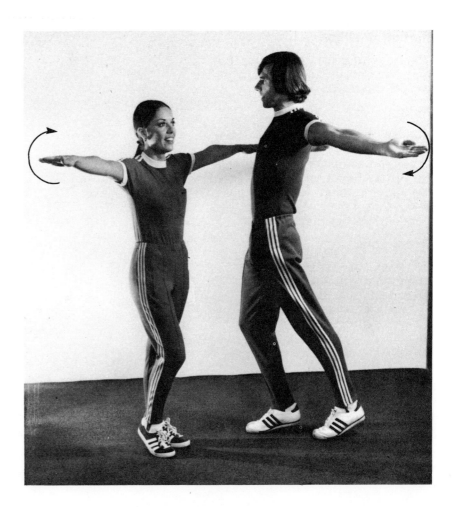

# EXERCISE 6   ARM ROWING*

## Starting Position

Walking erect, extend arms full length in front shoulder high, hands extended palms down.

## Action

Clench fists, pull arms back, bending elbows. Pull arms back, keeping elbows shoulder high, until fists are about level with chest. Then reach out to return to original position. With each extension or retraction take one step.

## Repetitions

Beginners     : 4 times
Intermediate : 8 times
Advanced      : 8 times

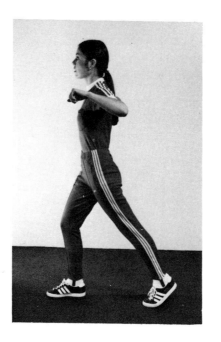
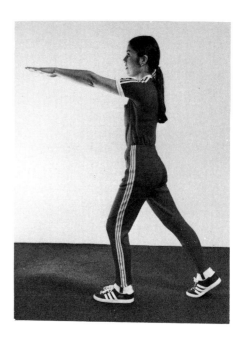

## EXERCISE 7   ARM SIDE EXTENSION*

### Starting Position

Walking erect, bend elbows shoulder high so that hands touch chest.

### Action

With first step extend arms out to the side shoulder high, letting arm swing back as far as possible. DO NOT LOWER ARMS. With second step return arms to original position across chest.

### Repetitions

Beginners    : 4 times
Intermediate : 8 times
Advanced     : 8 times

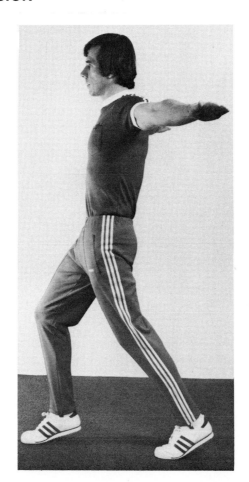
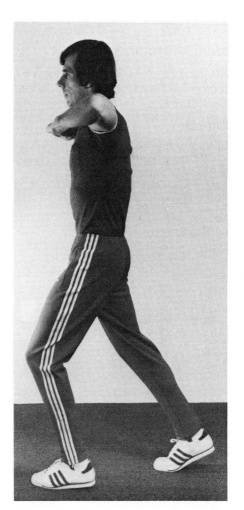

# EXERCISE 8   ALTERNATE FORWARD ARM THRUST

## Starting Position

Walking erect, left leg and right arm forward, left arm bent back shoulder high, fists clenched.

## Action

With each subsequent step the extended arm is pulled back and the bent arm is thrust forward.

## Duration

Beginners    : 4 times each arm
Intermediate : 6 times each arm
Advanced     : 8 times each arm

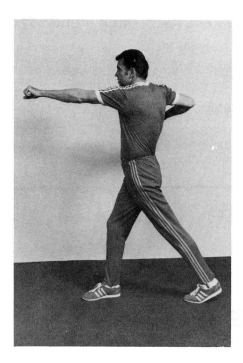

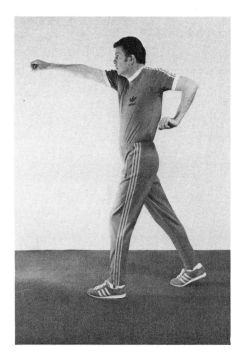

# EXERCISE 9   MARCHING BODY TWIST

## Starting Position

Body erect, hands clasped behind the head.

## Action

With each step twist the body toward the forward leg, bringing the elbow as far as possible to the front.

## Repetitions

Beginners    : 4 times each side
Intermediate : 6 times each side
Advanced     : 8 times each side

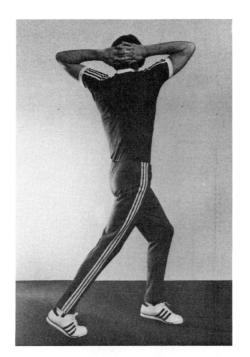

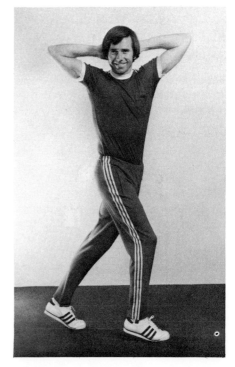

# EXERCISE 10   OVERHEAD ARM SWING

## Starting Position

Walking erect, arms hanging straight down at the sides.

## Action

With first step swing arms out front and over the head, keeping elbows straight. With second step lower arms to original position.

## Repetitions

Beginners    : 4 times
Intermediate : 6 times
Advanced     : 8 times

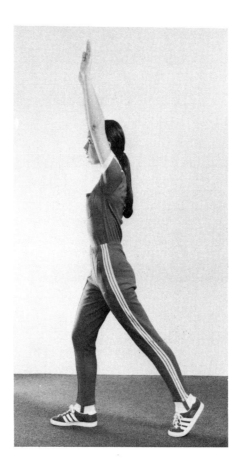
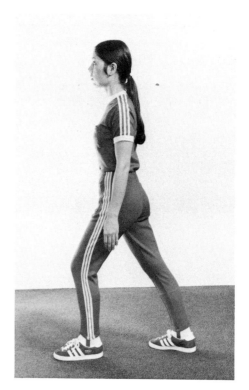

# EXERCISE 11   ANKLE GRASP

(not to be mistaken for a duckwalk)

## Starting Position

Grasp ankles with hands, keeping legs as sraight as possible. Force buttocks up.

## Action

Walk in a forward motion, keeping hands grasped around ankles. Keep buttocks up so that legs bend at knee as little as possible.

## Duration

Beginners     : 8–10 steps
Intermediate : 8–10 steps
Advanced      : 10–20 steps

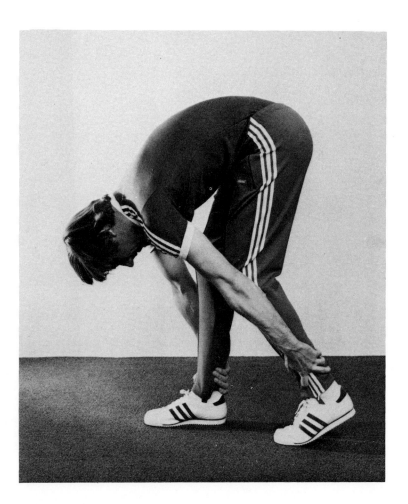

# EXERCISE 12   STRADDLE HOP

(Note: Exercises 12 to 18 are performed on the spot)

## Starting Position

Stand erect, feet together, hands on
hips.

## Action

On the first movement begin with a
slight jump spreading feet about 2
feet apart. On the second movement
return feet to original position.

## Repetitions

Beginners    : 4 times
Intermediate : 8 times
Advanced     : 8–10 times

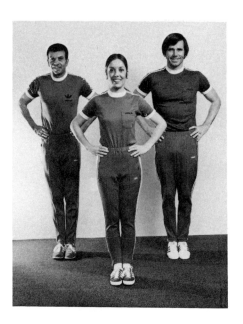
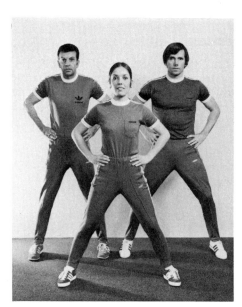

# EXERCISE 13   STRADDLE HOP—ARMS EXTENDED

## Starting Position

Stand erect, feet together, arms hanging straight down at sides.

## Action

On the first movement begin with a slight jump spreading feet about 2 feet apart. At the same time raise arms out to the sides shoulder high. On the second movement return feet and arms to original position.

## Repetitions

Beginners     : 4 times
Intermediate : 8 times
Advanced     : 8 times

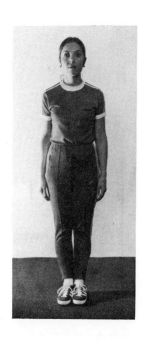

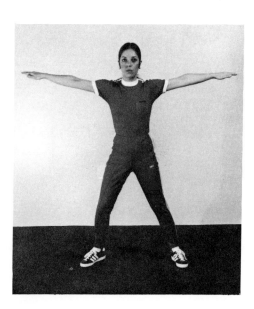

# EXERCISE 14   STRADDLE HOP—ARMS RAISED

## Starting Position

Stand erect, feet together, arms hanging straight down at sides.

## Action

On the first movement begin with a slight jump spreading feet about 2 feet apart. At the same time raise arms out to the sides and up over the head clapping hands. Keep arms as straight as possible. On the second movement return feet and arms to original position.

## Repetitions

Beginners : 4 times
Intermediate : 6 times
Advanced : 8–10 times

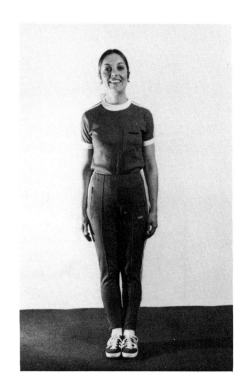
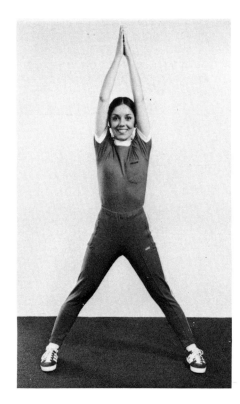

# EXERCISE 15 STRADDLE HOP—ARM AND LEG CROSSOVER

## Starting Position

Stand erect, feet 18 inches apart, arms extended to sides shoulder high.

## Action

On the first movement begin with a slight jump and cross legs, arms swing down and cross over in front of body. On second movement return feet and arms to original position.

Note: This exercise develops coordination.

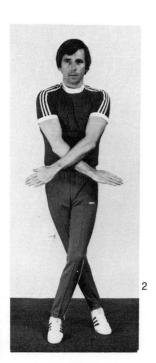

2

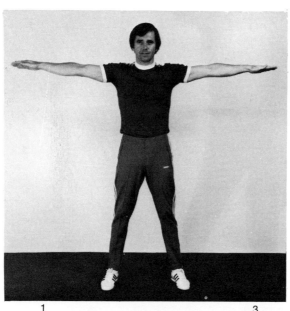

1

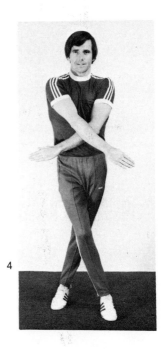

3

4

## Repetitions

Beginners     : None
Intermediate : 6 times
Advanced     : 8 times

# EXERCISE 16   FORWARD MOTION SIDE TO SIDE HOP

## Starting Position

Stand erect, feet together, hands on hips.

## Action

*Feet remain together throughout this exercise.* On first movement begin with a slight jump moving the feet forward and to the left. On second movement begin with a slight jump moving the feet back to the original position. On third movement move to the right as in first movement. Fourth movement is the same as the second. Repeat sequence.

Note:  This exercise is also good for Balance.

## Repetitions

Beginners    : None
Intermediate : 4 times each side
Advanced     : 8 times each side

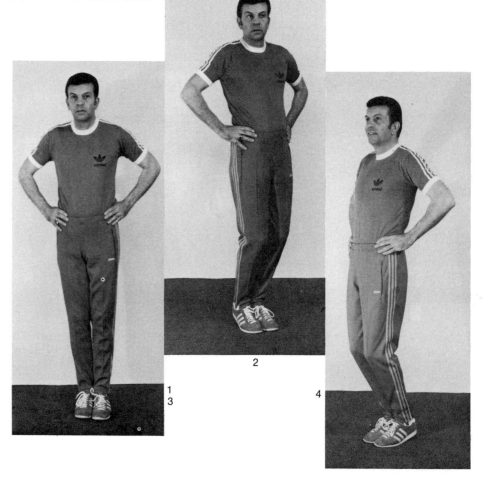

1
3

2

4

# EXERCISE 17   FRONT–BACK STRIDE HOP

## Starting Position

Stand erect, feet 18 inches apart, hands on hips.

## Action

On the first movement begin with a slight jump moving the legs forward about 1 foot, legs remain apart. On second movement legs move back from forward position about 2 feet. Hands remain on hips. On third movement legs move forward about 2 feet. Repeat second and third movements.

## Repetitions

Beginners    : 6 times
Intermediate : 8 times
Advanced     : 10 or more times

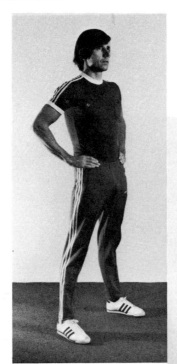
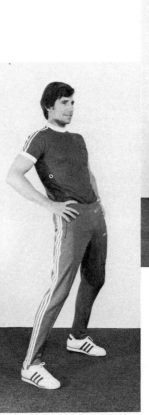
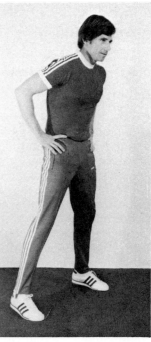

## EXERCISE 18 ~ FRONT-BACK STRIDE HOP WITH ARM RAISE

### Starting Position

Stand erect, feet 18 inches apart, hands hanging at sides.

### Action

On the first movement begin with a slight jump moving the legs forward about 1 foot keeping legs apart. At same time arms swing out in front and straight up over the head. On second movement legs move back from forward position about 2 feet and arms swing down to the sides. On third movement legs move forward about 2 feet and arms swing up over the head. Repeat second and third movements.

### Repetitions

Beginners    : None
Intermediate : 4–6 times
Advanced    : 8–10 times

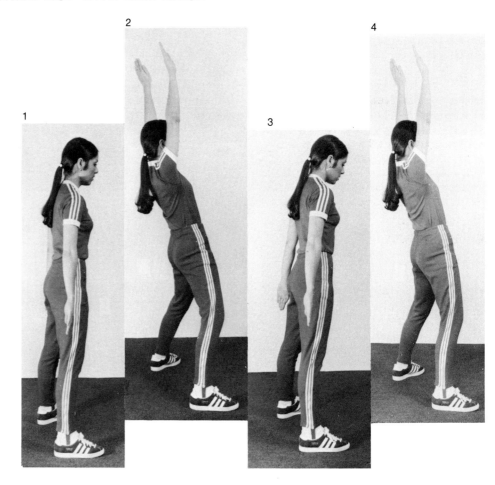

## EXERCISE 19 SIDE RUN

### Starting Position

Stand erect, knees slightly bent, feet together, hands on hips.

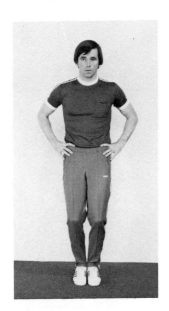

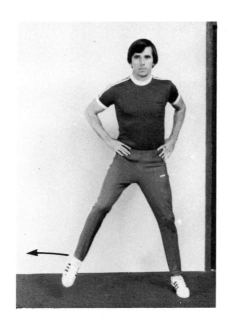

### Action

With a slightly bouncing motion move right leg about 18 inches to right, then bring left leg to right leg. Repeat sequence. Reverse movement to move left.

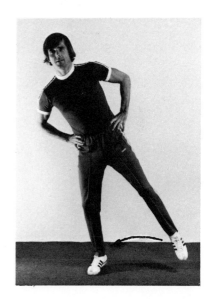

### Duration

Beginners : 10 times each way.
Intermediate : 15 times each way.
Advanced : 20-30 times each way.

## EXERCISE 20  SIDE RUN WITH ARM SWING

### Action

With a slightly bouncing motion move right leg about 18 inches to the right, at same time swinging arms out to sides shoulder high. Bring left leg to right leg, lower arms to sides and cross over slightly. Repeat sequence. Reverse movement to move left.

### Starting Position

Stand erect, feet together, hands at sides.

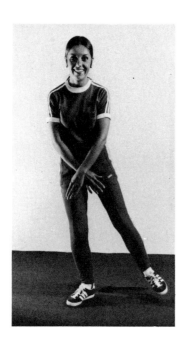

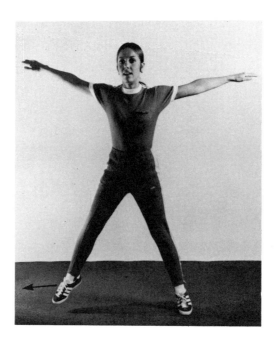

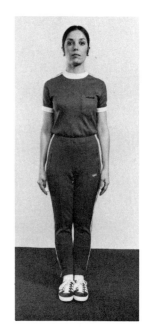

### Repetitions

Beginners     : 10 times each way
Intermediate : 15 times each way
Advanced    : 20-30 times each way.

## EXERCISE 21    SIDE RUN WITH LEG CROSSOVER

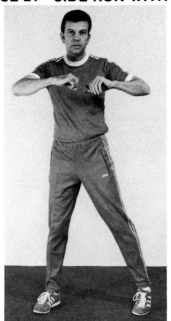
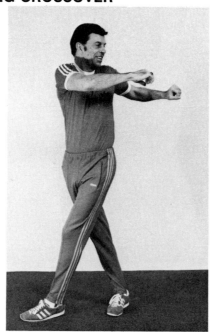
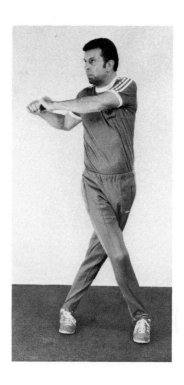

### Starting Position

Stand erect, feet together, hands at sides.

### Repetitions

Beginners : None
Intermediate : 10 times each way.
Advanced : 15–20 times each way.

### Action

With a slightly bouncing motion move right leg about 18 inches to the right. On second movement bring left leg across in front of right leg, turning lower body right and upper body left; arms swing left. On third movement bring right leg about 18 inches to right of left leg and straighten body. On fourth movement bring left leg across and behind right leg turning lower body left and upper body right; arms swing right. Repeat sequence. Reverse movement to move left.

# EXERCISE 22   HOPPING TORSO TWIST

## Starting Position

Stand with feet together, arms bent at elbows, knees slightly bent.

## Action

With a hopping motion, twist from side to side turning upper body and arms in opposite direction to feet.

## Repetitions

Beginners     : 5 times each way
Intermediate : 10 times each way
Advanced     : 15–20 times each way.

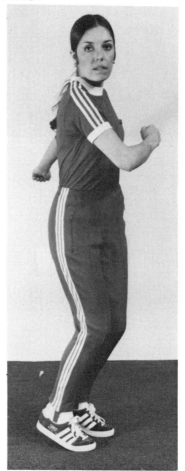
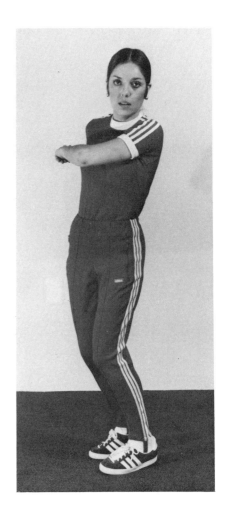

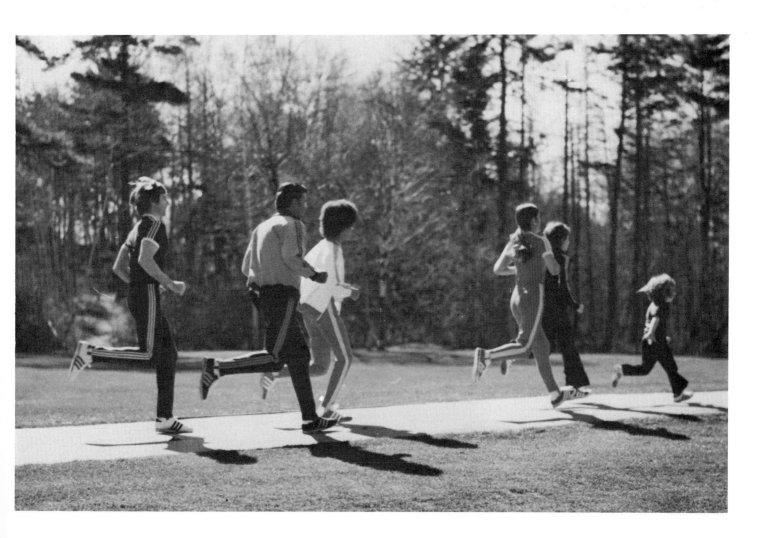

# The Loosen-Up

The loosen-up is designed specifically to gently exert the various muscle groups in the body.

As you have seen, many of the warm-up group of exercises also loosen up the body. The loosen-up group of exercises place special emphasis on those muscles that will be subjected to full stretching and pulling in the next section.

As in the warm-up period this group of exercises should be completed at a moderate pace.

The loosen-up period may also be extended to include any of the additional activities shown but must include those exercises designated with an asterisk.

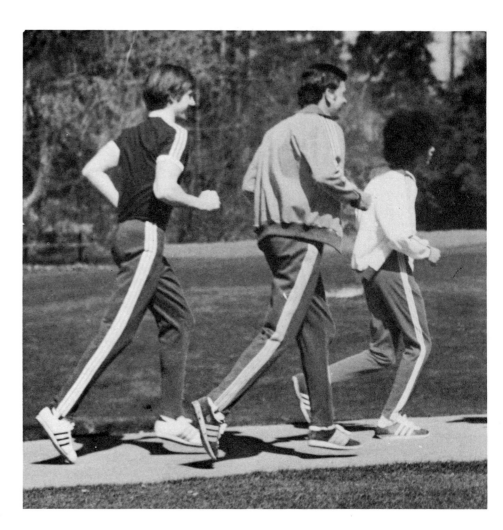

# EXERCISE 1  SHORT SIDE BEND*

## Starting Position

Stand erect, feet 1 foot to 18 inches apart, arms at the sides.

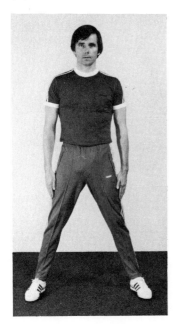

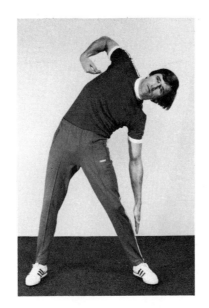

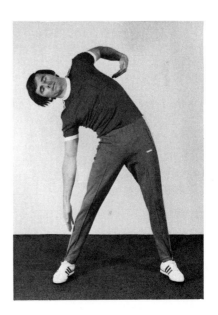

## Action

Keep the body at right angles to the floor; do not lean forward or backward. Keeping the feet firm on the floor, bend to the left, pulling left arm down to the side, tucking right hand up under right armpit. On second movement bend to right stretching right arm down to side tucking left hand up under left armpit. Repeat sequence.

## Repetitions

Beginners    : 8 times each side
Intermediate : 8 times each side
Advanced    : 8 times each side

# EXERCISE 2   SHORT SIDE BEND with ARM RAISE

## Starting Position

Stand erect, feet 1 foot to 18 inches apart, arms at the sides.

## Action

Keep the body at right angles to the floor, do not lean forward or backward. Keeping the feet firm on the floor, bend to the left, raising the right arm over the head and to the left side, pulling the left arm down to the side. On the second movement bend to right, raising the left arm over the head and to the right side, pulling the right arm down to the side. Repeat sequence.

## Repetitions

Beginners     : 4 times each side
Intermediate : 6 times each side
Advanced     : 8 times each side

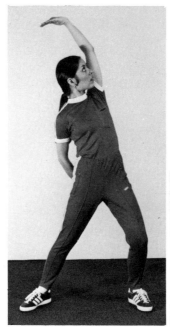
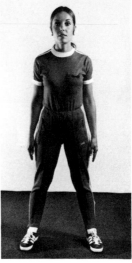
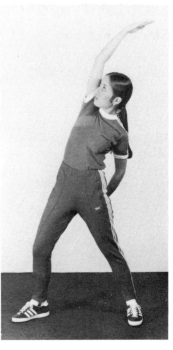

# EXERCISE 3  BODY TWIST—ARMS EXTENDED*

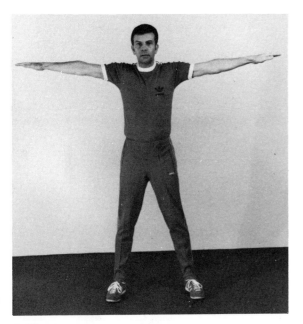

## Action

On the first movement twist the body to the left from the waist up, swinging the arms in the same direction. On the second movement twist the body all the way to the right keeping the arms extended at all times. DO NOT MOVE THE FEET. Repeat sequence.

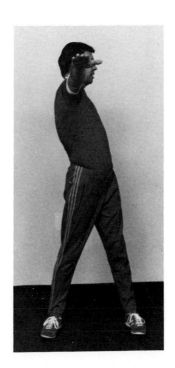

## Starting Position

Stand erect, feet 1 foot to 18 inches apart, arms extended out to the sides shoulder high.

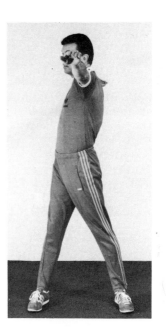

## Repetitions

Beginners      : 4 times each side
Intermediate : 8 times each side
Advanced     : 8 times each side

## EXERCISE 4 BODY TWIST—ARMS BENT*

(*Intermediate and Advanced)

### Starting Position

Stand erect, feet 1 foot to 18 inches apart, arms bent in toward chest shoulder high.

### Action

On the first movement twist the body to the left from the waist up; keep the arms bent, but pull the left shoulder back. On the second movement return left arm to original position, swing to the right, and pull the right shoulder back. Turn head in the direction you are pulling. Repeat sequence.

Unlike Exercise 3, this exercise places more strain on the shoulder group of muscles.

### Repetitions

Beginners : 4 times each side
Intermediate : 8 times each side
Advanced : 8 times each side

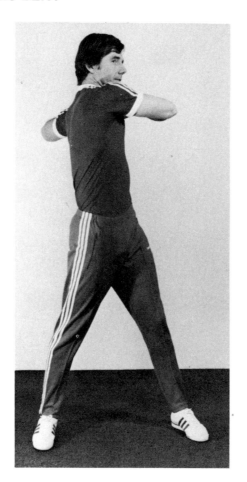
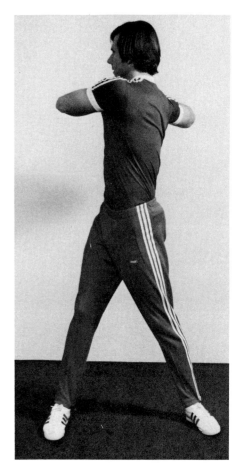

# EXERCISE 5   SINGLE SIDE ARM PULL

## Starting Position

Stand erect, feet together or 1 foot to 18 inches apart, arms bent in toward chest shoulder high.

## Action

On the first movement swing the left arm out and to the rear of the body as far as possible keeping the arm shoulder high. DO NOT TWIST THE BODY. On second movement, swing the left arm back to original position and the right arm out and to the rear of the body as far as possible keeping the arm shoulder high. Repeat sequence.

## Repetitions

Beginners     : 4 times each side
Intermediate : 6 times each side
Advanced     : 8 times each side

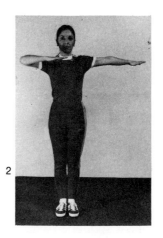

2

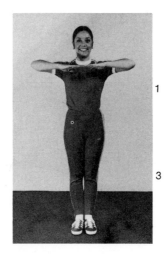

1

3

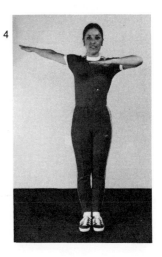

4

# EXERCISE 6   DOUBLE SIDE ARM PULL

## Starting Position

Stand erect, feet 1 foot to 18 inches apart, arms bent in toward chest shoulder high.

## Action

On the first movement swing both arms out and to the rear of the body as far as possible keeping arms shoulder high. It is permissible to raise up on the ball of the foot. On second movement return to original position. Repeat sequence.

## Repetitions

Beginners     : 4 times
Intermediate : 6 times
Advanced      : 8 times

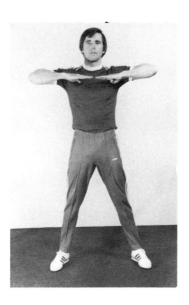
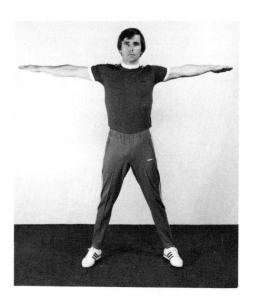

## EXERCISE 7   CROSSOVER TOE TOUCH*

### Starting Position

Stand erect, feet about 2 feet apart.
Hands hanging at sides.

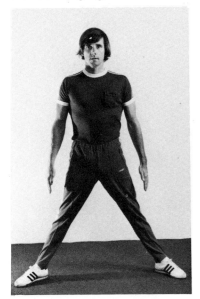

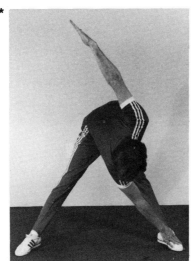

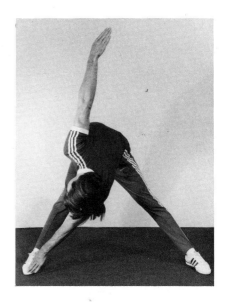

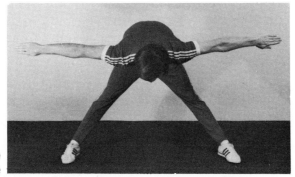

Note: alternate starting position

### Repetitions

Beginners : 4 times each side
Intermediate : 6 times each side
Advanced : 8 times each side

### Action

On first movement, swing right hand to left toe, bending body down and to the left at the waist. On second movement, return to original position and swing left hand to right toe. Repeat sequence. ON EACH MOVEMENT SWING FROM THE WAIST FIRST, THEN THE SHOULDER.

# EXERCISE 8  SHORT KNEE BEND

## Starting Position

Stand erect, toes 6 to 8 inches apart, heels together, arms hanging at sides.

## Action

Keeping heels together, raise up on ball of feet, swing arms out in front shoulder high, and bend knees about one-quarter of the way down. Keep back straight. On second movement, straighten knees, lower arms and heels. Repeat sequence.

## Repetitions

Beginners     : 4 times
Intermediate : 6 times
Advanced     : 8 times

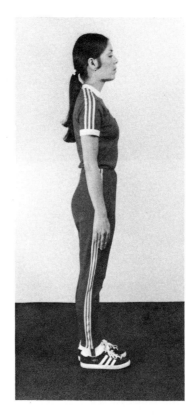
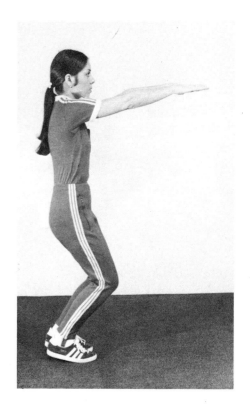

# EXERCISE 9  DOUBLE TOE TOUCH—SHOULDER PULL

## Starting Position

This exercise can be done feet to-gether or apart. If feet apart they should be about 18 inches.

## Action

On first movement bend forward from the waist and touch toes (Note: Bend the waist first then the shoul-ders.). On second movement straighten up, bend arms, and pull arms back shoulder high. Repeat sequence.

## Repetitions

Beginners    : 4 times
Intermediate : 6 times
Advanced     : 8 times

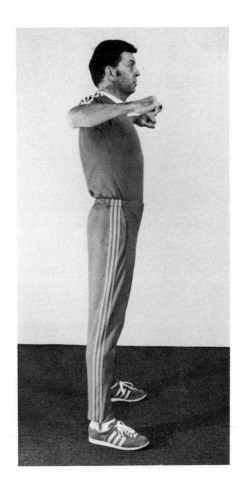
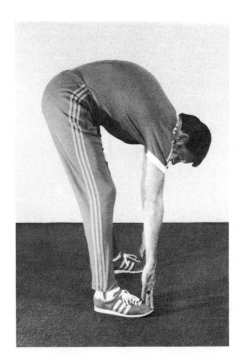

# EXERCISE 10  DOUBLE TOE TOUCH—OVERHEAD ARM EXTENSION

## Starting Position

This exercise can be done feet to-gether or apart. If feet apart they should be about 18 inches. Arms hang at sides.

## Action

On first movement bend forward from the waist, touch toes (Note: Bend the waist first then the shoulders.). On second movement straighten up and raise arms straight up over head. Repeat sequence.

## Repetitions

Beginners    : None
Intermediate : 4 times
Advanced     : 8 times

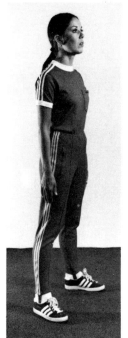
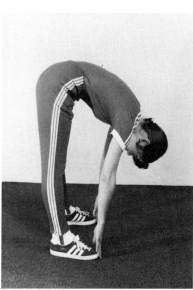
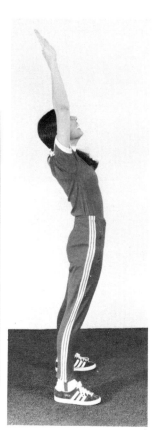

# EXERCISE 11   SITTING CROSSOVER TOE TOUCH*

## Starting Position

Sit on floor, legs in front, feet about 2 to 3 feet apart.
(Note: In this exercise it is permissible to bend the knees slightly.)

## Action

Reach right hand over, bending the waist forward and turning the upper body left. Touch left toe. On second movement twist the waist right and reach for right toe with left hand. Free arm should swing to back.

## Repetitions

Beginners    : 4 times each side
Intermediate : 4 times each side
Advanced     : 8 times each side

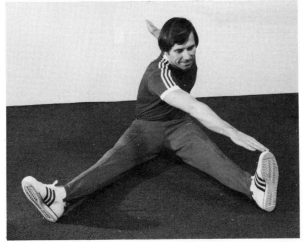

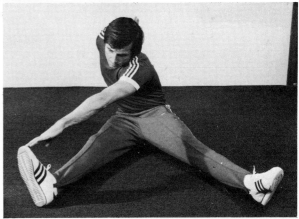

# EXERCISE 12   SITTING DOUBLE TOE TOUCH—OVERHEAD ARM EXTENSION

## Starting Position

Sit on floor, legs in front, feet about 2 to 3 feet apart.

(Note: In this exercise it is permissible to bend the knees slightly.)

## Action

Reach out to toes with both hands, bending from waist, then sit up straight raising arms over head in a side swinging motion. Clap hands overhead keeping arms straight. Repeat.

## Repetitions

Beginners    : 4 times
Intermediate : 6 times
Advanced     : 8 times

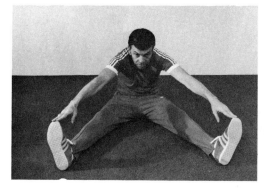
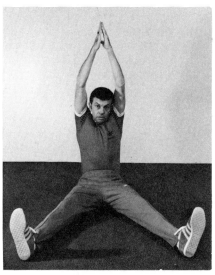

## EXERCISE 13   SITTING ARM STRETCH—OVERHEAD ARM EXTENSION

### Starting Position

Sit on floor, legs in front, feet about
2 to 3 feet apart.
(Note: In this exercise it is permis-
         sible to bend the knees
         slightly.)

### Action

Keeping hands together, reach as
far in front as possible to touch
hands to floor, then sit up straight
raising arms overhead in a side
swinging motion. Clap hands overhead keeping arms straight. Repeat.

### Repetitions

Beginners    : None
Intermediate : 4 times
Advanced     : 8 times

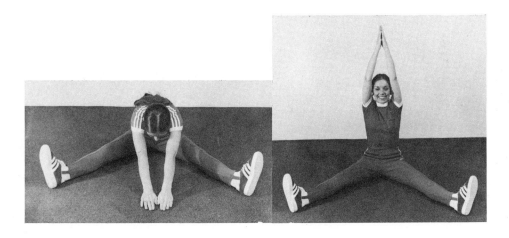

## EXERCISE 14    MID-TORSO RAISE

### Starting Position

Sit on floor, legs out front, feet together or about 8 to 10 inches apart. Hands on floor about 1 foot behind shoulders elbows straight.

### Action

From sitting position, swing mid-section up as far as possible by arching back, leaving only hands and feet on floor. Let head rock back. On second movement return to original position. Repeat.

### Repetitions

Beginners     : 4 times
Intermediate : 6 times
Advanced     : 8 times

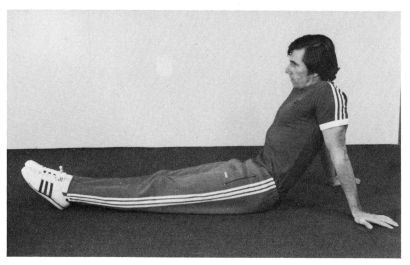

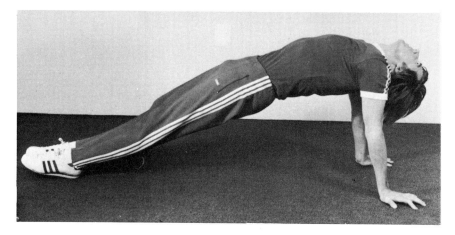

# EXERCISE 15  EXTENDED LEG RAISE

## Starting Position

Sit on floor, legs out front, feet about 8 to 10 inches apart. Hands on floor about 1 foot behind shoulders, elbows straight.

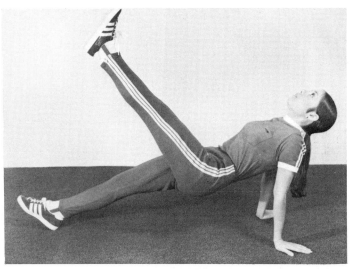

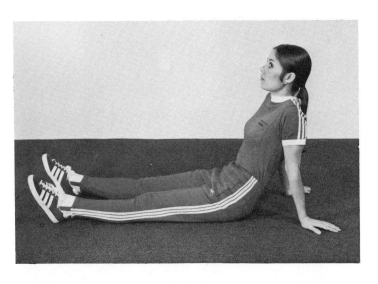

## Action

From sitting position raise mid-section up until body is in a prone position. At the same time kick left leg up as far as possible. Lower body and leg at same time. Reverse and repeat sequence.

## Repetitions

Beginners    : None
Intermediate : 4 times
Advanced     : 8 times

# EXERCISE 16 CROSSOVER LEG STRETCH

## Starting Position

Sit on floor, legs out front, feet together. Hands on floor slightly behind shoulders, elbows straight.

## Action

From sitting position, raise right leg and cross over left leg. Lower leg, toe to touch floor as high above the middle section as possible. Keep knee straight. Return to original position and reverse. Repeat sequence.

## Repetitions

Beginners : 4 times each side
Intermediate : 6 times each side
Advanced : 8 times each side

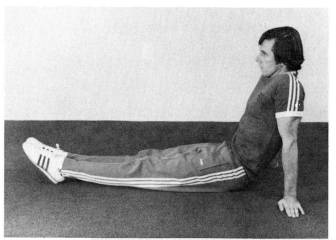

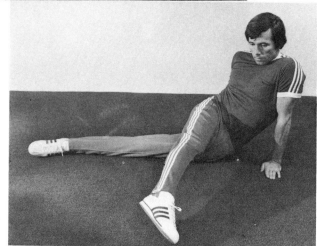

# EXERCISE 17   FRONT KICK—HAND CLAP

## Starting Position

Stand erect, feet together, hands extended shoulder high at sides.

## Action

Kick right leg up in front as high as possible. Clap hands under right leg. Lower right leg and swing hands to the sides shoulder high. Kick left leg up in front as high as possible and repeat remainder of exercise as before. Repeat sequence.

*Note:* This exercise also develops Balance

## Repetitions

Beginners    : None
Intermediate : 4 times each leg
Advanced     : 6 times each leg

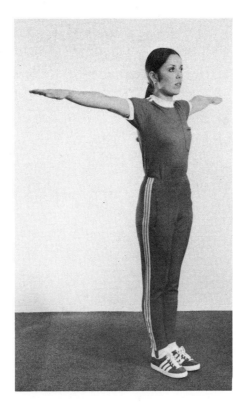
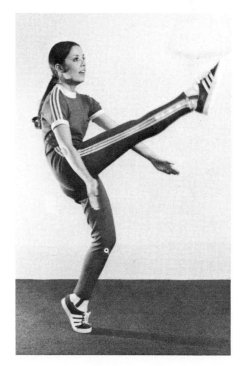

# Stretching, Bending, Pulling

This portion of the exercise program is designed to exert the various muscle groups in the body. If done properly, these exercises should cause even the conditioned athlete to strain the muscle groups. These exercises are a natural extension of the loosen-up group and are in actual fact the beginning of the muscle conditioning program.

In these exercises the pace is moderate to slow. Emphasis should be placed in getting the full reach, bend, or pull from the exercise. It is important to get a full bend or twist at a slow pace rather than a half bend at a fast pace.

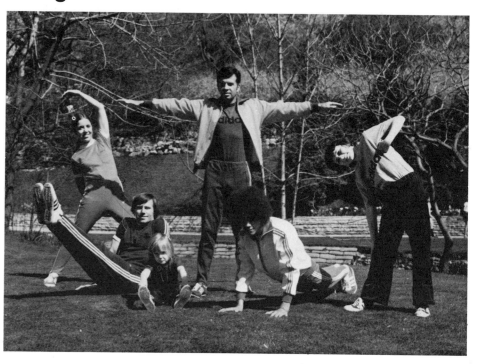

# EXERCISE 1   DEEP SIDE BEND

## Starting Position

Stand erect, feet together, hands at sides.

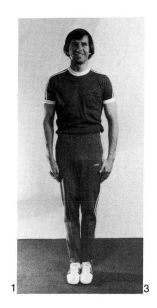

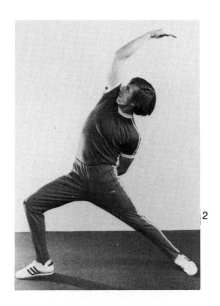

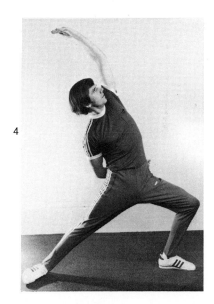

## Repetitions

Beginners    : 2 times each side
Intermediate : 3 times each side
Advanced     : 5 times each side

## Action

Step out with right leg, bend knee, bend waist to the left. Swing left arm to the back and right, right arm to the left over the head. Pull to count of three. Return to original position and repeat stepping to left. Repeat sequence.

## EXERCISE 2   DEEP KNEE BEND

NOTE: This exercise can be harmful
to the knees and should only
be done by persons who are
NOT overweight and who are
in good physical condition.

### Starting Position

Stand erect, feet together, hands at
sides.

### Action

Raise up on ball of feet, raise arms
straight out in front shoulder high.
Keeping back straight assume a low
squat position. Stand up; lower
arms as rest back of feet. Repeat
sequence.

### Repetitions

Beginners    : None
Intermediate : None
Advanced     : 4 times

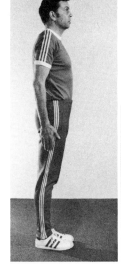
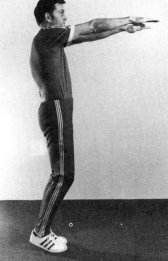
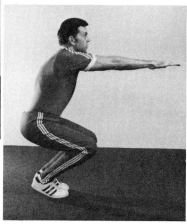

## EXERCISE 3  BURPEES

Note: This exercise can also be harmful to the knees. Be sure to push off the floor with the hands to take some of the weight of the body off the knees.

### Starting Position

Stand erect, feet together, hands at sides.

### Action

Take a small jump on the spot; land on balls of feet, knees slightly bent, and immediately squat placing hands palms down on the floor. Kick both legs straight back. Bend both legs to chest. With a slight jump, pushing off the floor with the hands stand up straight and let arms return to the sides. Repeat sequence.

### Repetitions

Beginners    : None
Intermediate : 2 times
Advanced     : 4 times

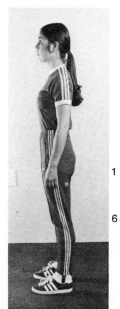

1

6

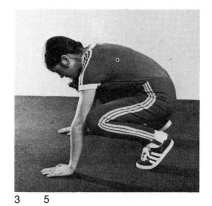

2

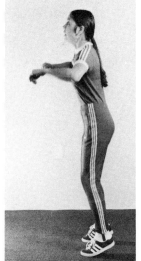

3   5

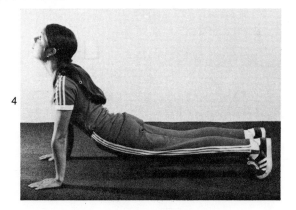

4

# EXERCISE 4   ALTERNATE LEG BURPEES

### Starting Position

Stand erect, feet together, hands at sides.

### Action

Squat to floor, placing hands palms down on floor. Keeping right leg bent, kick left leg straight back. Bend left leg to chest. Pushing off with hands stand up straight and let arms return to the sides. Repeat sequence extending right leg to rear.

### Repetitions

Beginners    : None
Intermediate : 2 times each leg
Intermediate : 4 times each leg

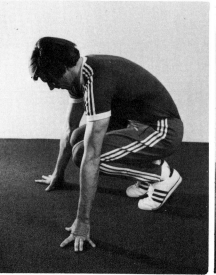

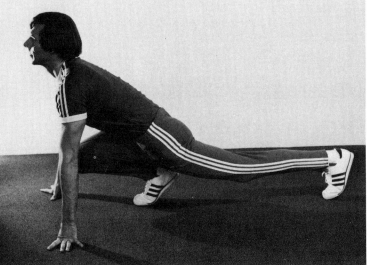

# EXERCISE 5   ANKLE GRASP AND PULL

## Starting Position

Stand erect, feet together, hands at sides.

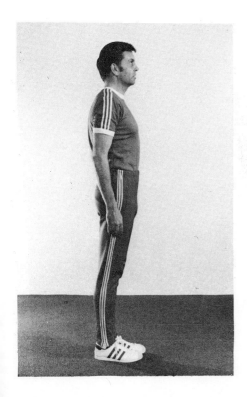

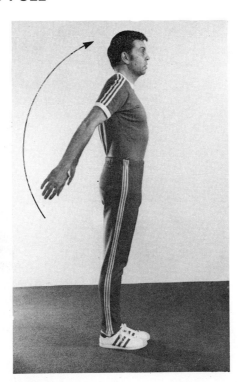

## Action

Swing arms to rear and up over head. Bending from waist, swing arms down and grasp ankles. Pull down three times and return to starting position. Repeat sequence.

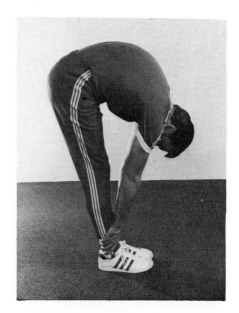

## Repetitions

Beginners     : 2 times
Intermediate : 3 times
Advanced     : 4 times

# EXERCISE 6  DEEP STRETCH AND TWIST

## Starting Position

Stand erect, feet apart, hands together overhead, elbows straight.

## Action

Twist body to right, bend down and touch right toes, then touch floor in centre between feet. Twist to left side touch left toes and straighten up, raising arms up over head. Repeat sequence, then reverse sequence going from left to right.

## Repetitions

Beginners     : 4 times each direction
Intermediate : 6 times each direction
Advanced     : 8 times each direction

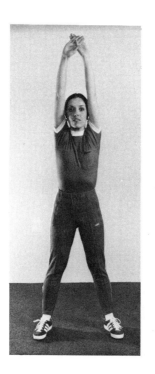
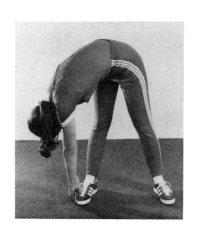
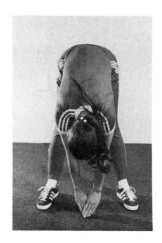
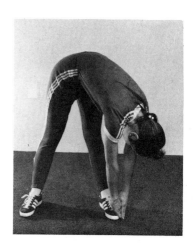

# EXERCISE 7   TOE TOUCH—ARM SWING

## Starting Position

Stand erect, feet apart, arms straight out in front shoulder high.

## Action

Swing arms in a wide circle to rear and over head twice. On second swing bend forward at waist and touch floor in between legs and then touch toes. Straighten up and repeat sequence.

## Repetitions

Beginners     : 4 times
Intermediate : 6 times
Advanced      : 8 times

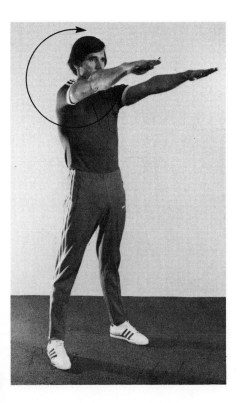

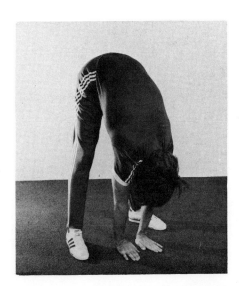

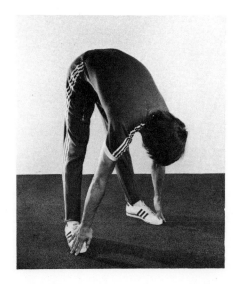

# EXERCISE 8   ALTERNATE TOE TOUCH—OVERHEAD ARM EXTENSION

## Starting Position

Stand erect, feet apart, arms straight up over the head.

## Action

Keeping arms extended, bend at waist and touch right toes. Straighten up (arms over head), bend at waist and touch left toes. Repeat sequence.

## Repetitions

Beginners     : 2 times each side
Intermediate : 4 times each side
Advanced     : 6–8 times each side

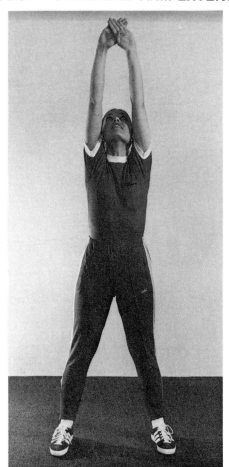

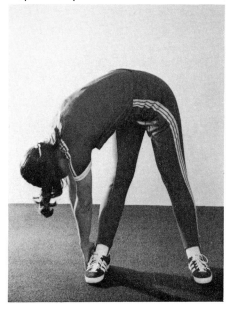

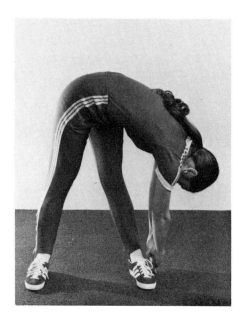

# EXERCISE 9  ALTERNATE HEEL TOUCH—OVERHEAD ARM EXTENSION

## Starting Position

Stand erect, feet together, arms straight up over head.

## Action

Keeping arms extended, squat, twist at waist to left, and touch left heel. Straighten up (arms over head) and repeat to right heel. Repeat sequence.

## Repetitions

Beginners     : None
Intermediate : 2 times each side
Advanced     : 4 times each side

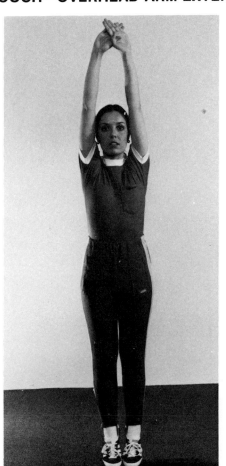

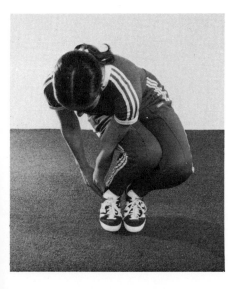

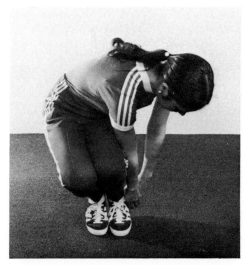

# EXERCISE 10   ROTATING WAIST BEND

## Starting Position

Place hands on hips, feet apart, and bend forward at the waist.

## Action

Rotate upper body from the waist up in a clockwise motion. Repeat and then reverse rotation direction.

## Repetitions

Beginners      : 4 times each direc-
                                     tion
Intermediate : 6 times each direc-
                                     tion
Advanced     : 8 times each direc-
                                     tion

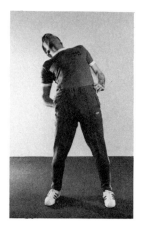
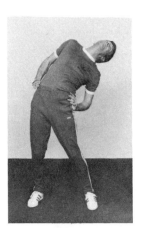
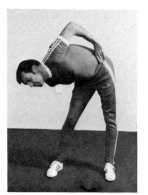
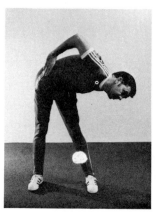
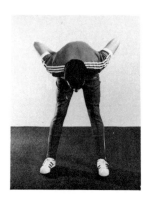

## EXERCISE 11  SINGLE SIDE LEG RAISE

### Starting Position

Lie on left side, right hand on hip, left arm on floor.

### Action

Raise right leg pointing toe in direction of head, reach up with right hand, and touch toes. Leg should be raised at right angle to body. Lower leg and arm. Repeat sequence on right side.

### Repetitions

Beginners    : 4 times on each side
Intermediate : 6 times on each side
Advanced     : 8 times on each side

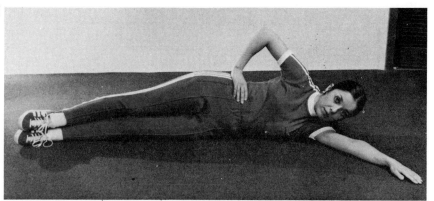

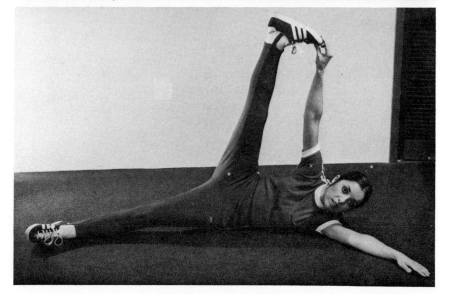

## EXERCISE 12   DOUBLE SIDE LEG RAISE

### Starting Position

Lie on left side, right hand on hip, left arm on floor.

### Action

Keeping right hand on hip raise both legs 8 to 10 inches off the ground. At same time raise upper body 8 to 10 inches off ground. Do NOT allow body to twist. Lower body to original position. Repeat sequence on right side.

### Repetitions

Beginners     : 4 times on each side
Intermediate : 6 times on each side
Advanced     : 8 times on each side

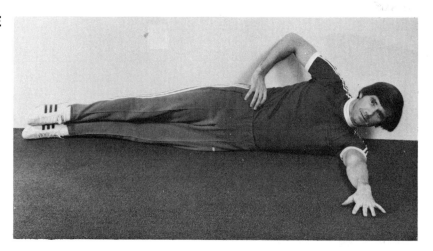

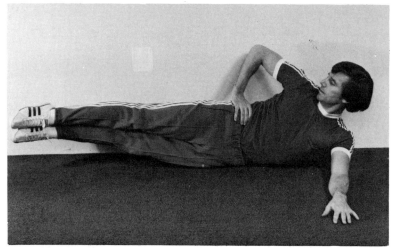

## EXERCISE 13   EXTENDED ARM RAISE

### Starting Position

Lie on stomach, arms outstretched over head, hands on floor.

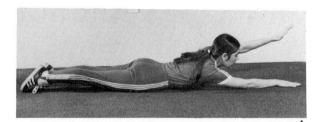

Starting Position

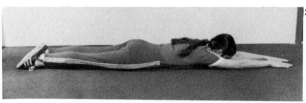

A

### Repetitions

Beginners     : 4 times each side
Intermediate : 6 times each side
Advanced     : 8 times each side

### Action

There are a number of simple variations to this exercise:

a) raise left arm as high as possible keeping arm over head at all times. Repeat and reverse.

b) Raise right arm, swinging it slightly to side, then swing it back as far as possible. Repeat and reverse.

c) Raise both arms at same time keeping arms overhead. Repeat.

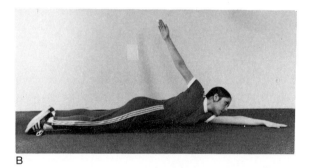

B

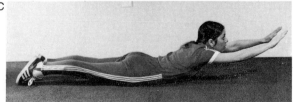

C

# EXERCISE 14  EXTENDED LEG RAISE

## Starting Position

Lie on stomach, arms bent at sides, hands palms down at shoulders.

## Action

Raise right leg as high as possible, arching back, but do not bend leg at knee. Lower leg and raise left in same manner. Repeat sequence.

## Repetitions

Beginners     : 4 times each leg
Intermediate : 6 times each leg
Advanced     : 8 times each leg

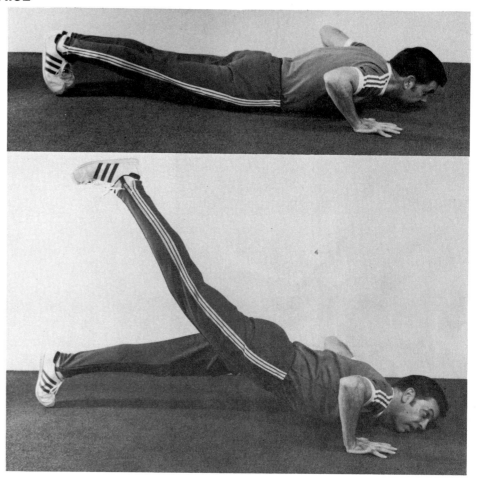

## EXERCISE 15   BACK ARCH

### Starting Position

Lie on stomach,
a) hands clasped at small of back,
   or

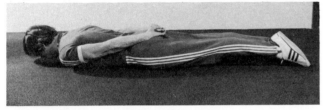

b) hands clasped behind head.

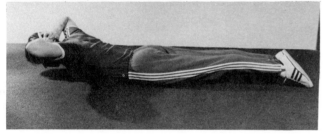

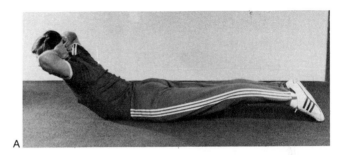

A

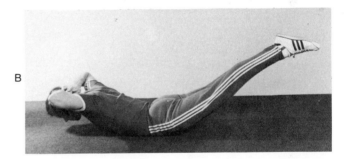

B

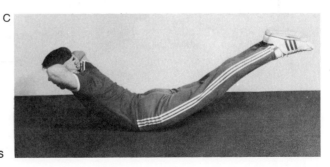

C

### Action

Lift upper body from waist, as high as possible and lower. Repeat. This exercise can also be done raising both legs, by rocking from waist, or by raising upper body and legs.

### Repetitions

Beginners    : None
Intermediate : 4 times
Advanced     : 6–8 times

# EXERCISE 16  BACK ARCH WITH ANKLE GRASP

## Starting Position

Lie on stomach and grasp ankles from back with hands.

## Action

Arch upper body and pull on ankles at the same time. Then relax keeping hold of ankles. Repeat.

## Repetitions

Beginners    : None
Intermediate : 4 times
Advanced     : 6–8 times

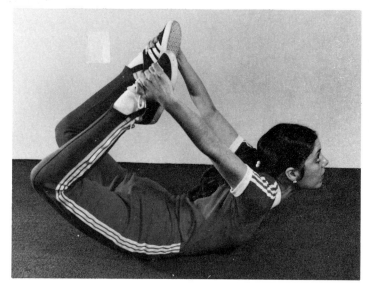

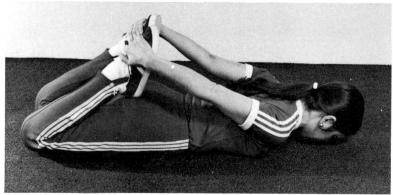

## EXERCISE 17   TORSO BENDS—ELBOWS

### Starting Position

Lie on stomach, resting upper body on elbows and forearm.

### Action

Raise seat as high as possible and lower to floor. Repeat.

### Repetitions

Beginners     : 4 times
Intermediate : 6 times
Advanced     : 8 times

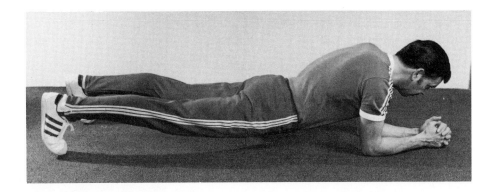

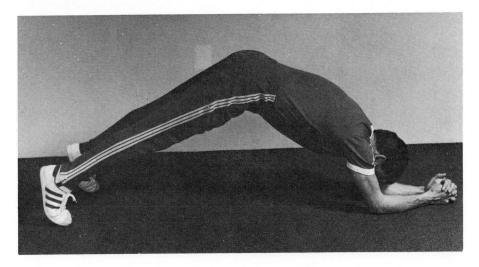

## EXERCISE 18   TORSO BENDS—FULL EXTENSION

### Starting Position

Lie on stomach, arms at full extension, palms on floor.

### Action

Raise seat as high as possible and lower to floor. Repeat.

### Repetitions

Beginners     : None
Intermediate : 4 times
Advanced     : 8 times

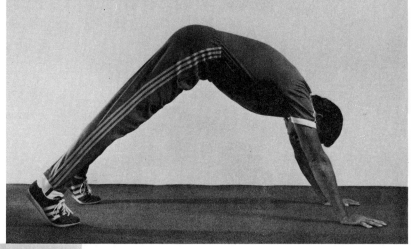

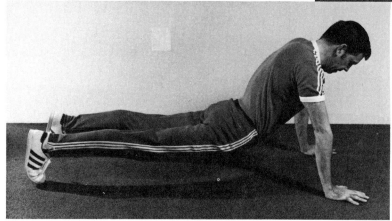

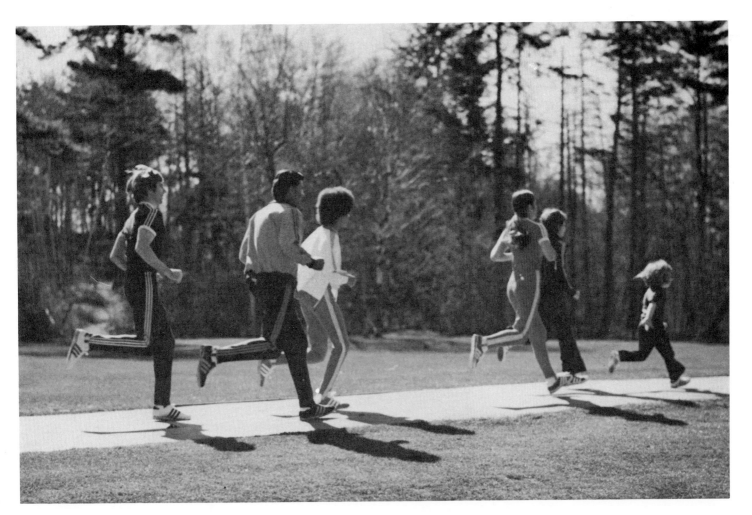

79

# Muscle Toning

This portion of the program is designed to condition the muscles. If done properly, these exercises will strengthen the muscles, not *build* them as in weight training. Even so, if muscles are not the size they should be for your bone structure, these exercises will build the exerted muscles.

The pace is moderate in the Muscle Toning exercises: the emphasis should be placed on getting the full extension out of each movement.

## CAUTION NOTES

### Push-Up Exercises

At all times when doing a full push-up or any of its variations, be sure to keep the back straight. Do *not* allow the back to sway down with a bouncing motion.

### Sit-Up and V-Sit Exercises

When doing these exercises the upper body is raised in a rolling motion; lift the head, shoulders, chest, and then the stomach as indicated. *Do not* try to lift the back straight—it can cause undue back strain. The rolling motion is easier on the back and the stomach works harder.

Sitting on a small foam pad is an excellent idea and prevents bruising of the tailbone during the sit-up portion of the program. It does not, however, make the exercises any easier.

*Do not* place the feet under any object that will hold them down. It is much safer to allow the feet to raise off the floor until the muscles are sufficiently conditioned to enable your feet to remain on the floor without aid.

When you can perform 8 to 10 sit-ups without lifting the feet off the ground, it is considered safe to use an aid to hold feet on the ground for rapid succession repetitions. If necessary, permit the knees to bend slightly; however, try to keep them as straight as possible.

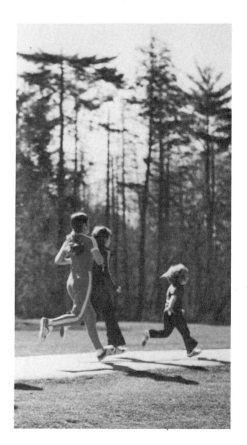

## EXERCISE 1   WAIST PUSH-UP

### Starting Position

Lie on stomach, feet together, hands on floor at shoulders.

*Note:* This exercise can be done with palms up or palms down. the palms-up version helps strengthen the wrists. It can also be done with fingers touching.

### Action

Bending from the waist, bring arms to a full extension and bend head back. Bending arms, lower body to original position. Repeat.

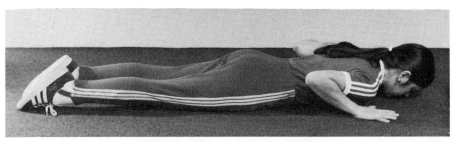

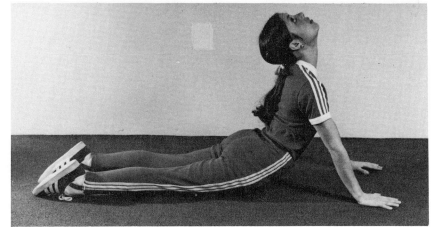

Hand Positions

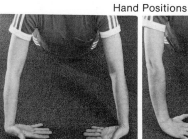 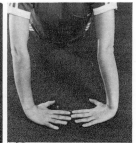

### Repetitions

Beginners      : 4 times
Intermediate : 8 times
Advanced     : 8 times

## EXERCISE 2   HALF PUSH-UP

### Starting Position

Lie on stomach, feet together. Bend legs at right angles to body. Hands on floor at shoulders.
*Note:* Can also be done palms up or down.

### Action

Pivoting from knees, bring arms to full extension and bend head back. Bending arms, lower body to original position. Repeat.

### Repetitions

Beginners    : 4 times
Intermediate : 6 times
Advanced     : 8 times

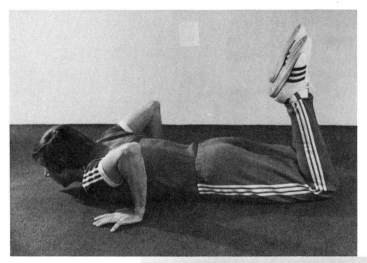

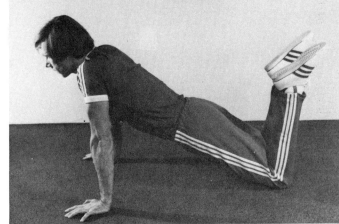

## EXERCISE 3   FULL PUSH-UP

### Starting Position

Lie on stomach, legs at full extension. Hands at shoulders, palms down.

*Note:* See variations on following pages.

### Action

Keeping back straight, raise body up by straightening arms. Lower body by bending arms. Repeat.

*Note:* Body should not rest on floor after each push-up, but rather be 3 to 4 inches off ground to retain tension.

### Repetitions

Beginners    : 2–4 times
Intermediate : 6 times
Advanced     : 8 times

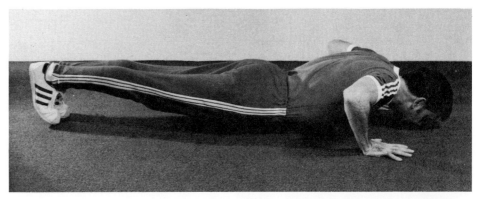

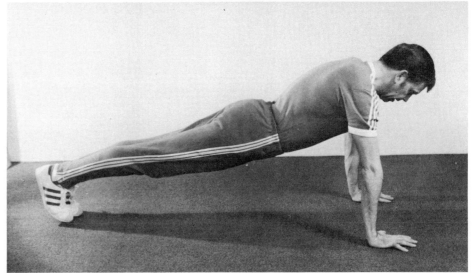

## VARIATIONS OF FULL PUSH-UP

*Note:* These variations should not be tried until you have mastered the regular push-up.

1. Cross right leg over left.

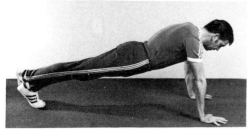

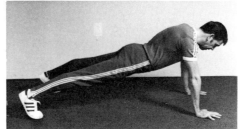

3. Spread feet apart.

4. Place hands together, fingers touching.

5. Place hands far apart.

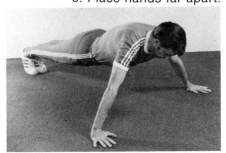

2. Cross left leg over right.

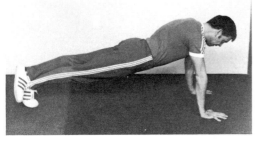

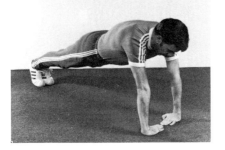

6. Clap hands.

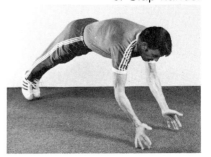

## EXERCISE 4   EXTENDED PUSH-UP

### Starting Position

Lie on stomach, legs at full extension, arms at full extension above
the head, palms down.

### Action

Raise body off the floor using the
toes and hands as support. When
lifting the body the first action is to
stiffen the body then lift. *Do not use
elbows or knees to assist in lift.*
Repeat.
*Note:* Women may use forearm.

### Repetitions

Beginners    : None
Intermediate : None
Advanced     : 2–4 times.

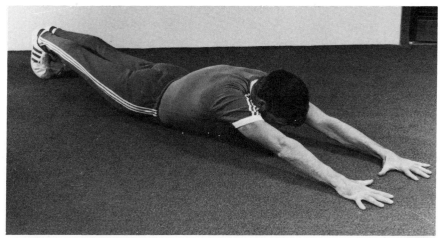

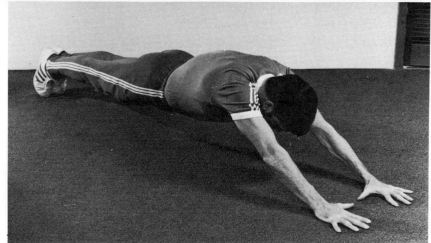

## EXERCISE 5 PUSH-UP—FOUR COUNT

### Starting Position

Lie on stomach, legs at full extension. Hands at shoulders, palms down.

### Action

Keeping back straight, raise body up by straightening arms. When arms at full extension, bend at waist pulling seat up as far as possible. Lower seat until body straight, then lower body by bending arms. Repeat.

*Note:* Body should not rest on floor after each push-up, but rather be 3 to 4 inches off ground to retain tension.

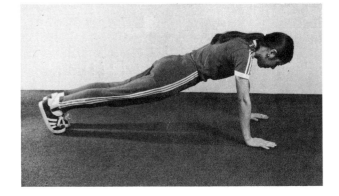

### Repetitions

Beginners    : None
Intermediate : 4 times
Advanced     : 8 times

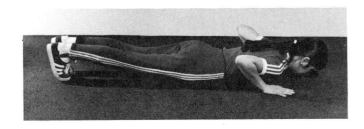

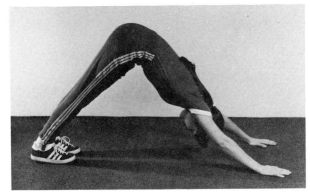

# EXERCISE 6   PUSH-UP—EIGHT COUNT

## Starting Position

Place body and stomach down to floor, hands at shoulders, arms at full extension.

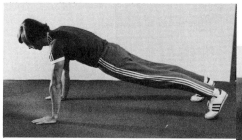

6

## Action

Lower body to within 3 to 4 inches of floor, then straighten elbows to raise body. When arms at full extension, bend at waist pulling seat up as far as possible. Lower body in a forward motion by pulling it down

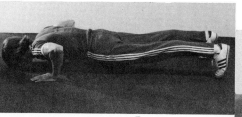

1   7   2

between arms and swinging up until body once again is straight and arms at full extension. Lower body to within 3 to 4 inches of floor then straighten elbows to raise body. Repeat sequence.

## Repetitions

Beginners : None
Intermediate : None
Advanced : 4–8 times

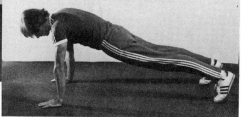

8

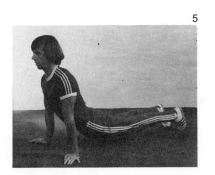

5

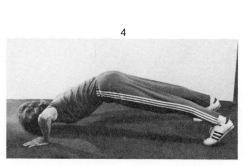

4

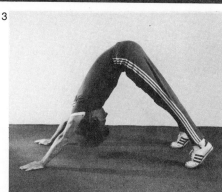

3

# EXERCISE 7  BODY PULL THROUGH

## Starting Position

Place body and stomach down to floor, hands at shoulders, arms at full extension, seat arched as high as possible.

## Action

Lower body in a forward motion by pulling it down between arms, swinging up and back until seat is once again arched as high as possible. Repeat.

## Repetitions

Beginners    : None
Intermediate : 2–4 times
Advanced    : Sets of 8

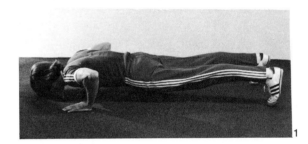

1

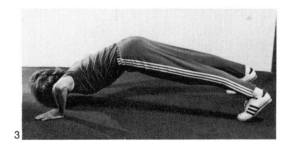

3

2

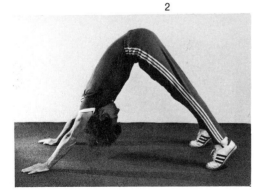

4

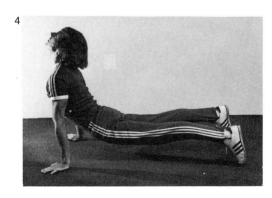

## EXERCISE 8   SIDE PUSH-UP

### Starting Position

Lie on floor on right side, left hand on hip, right arm fully extended, hand on floor palm down. Keep body curved at waist.
*Note:* Same exercise can be done on left side.

### Action

Arm does not bend. Raise body at waist as high as possible. Lower to starting position. Repeat.

### Repetitions

Beginners     : None
Intermediate : 6 times each side
Advanced     : 8 times each side

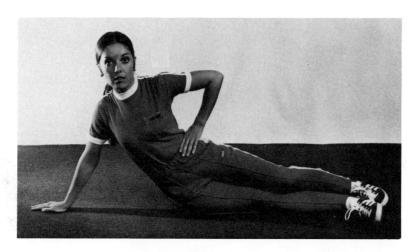

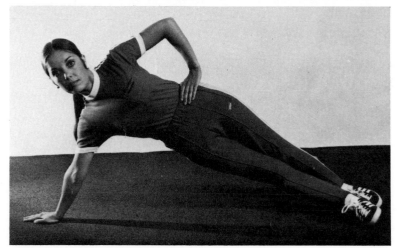

# EXERCISE 9   SIDE PUSH-UP WITH LEG RAISE

## Starting Position

Lie on floor on right side, left hand on hip, right arm fully extended hand on floor palm down. Keep body curved at waist.

*Note:* Same exercise can be done on left side.

## Action

Arm does not bend. Raise body at waist as high as possible. At same time raise left leg at right angles to the body. Lower body to starting position and lower leg. Repeat sequence.

## Repetitions

Beginners    : None
Intermediate : 4 times each side
Advanced     : 8 times each side

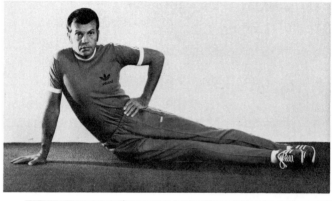

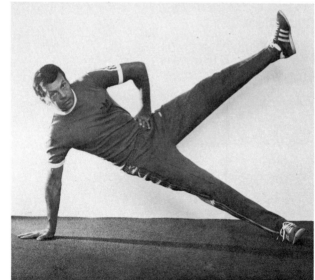

# EXERCISE 10   SIT-UP WITH FULL EXTENSION

## Starting Position

Lie on back on floor, legs spread apart, arms extended over the head.

## Action

Raise arms and upper body in rolling motion and reach down and touch toes. Keeping feet on floor, return to starting position. Repeat.

## Repetitions

Beginners    : 4 times
Intermediate : 8 times
Advanced     : 8 times

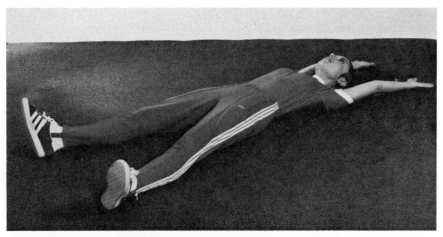

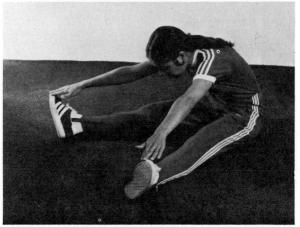

# EXERCISE 11   SIT-UP WITH LEG GRASP

## Starting Position

Lie on back, legs spread apart, arms extended to sides.

*Note:* Exercise may also be done keeping feet 4 to 6 inches off ground at beginning and end of exercise, but for *advanced only.*

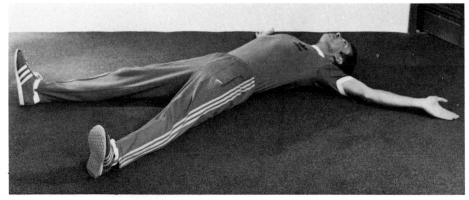

## Action

Swing arms to front and raise upper and lower body at waist bending knees to chest. Grasp legs below knees and squeeze to chest. Lower upper and lower body to original position and extend arms to sides. Repeat.

## Repetitions

Beginners     : 4 times
Intermediate : 6 times
Advanced     : 8 times

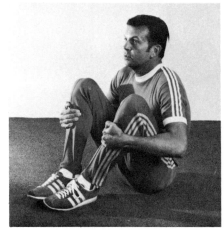

# EXERCISE 12   SIT-UP WITH HANDS BEHIND HEAD

## Starting Position

Lie on back, legs spread apart, arms folded, hands clasped behind head.

## Action

Raise body in rolling motion from waist and reach down as far as possible to touch knees with elbows. Lower body in rolling motion to original position. Repeat.

*Note:* Exercise may also be done crossing one elbow over to opposite knee and then the other before lowering body.

## Repetitions

Beginners    : None
Intermediate : 4 times
Advanced     : 8 times

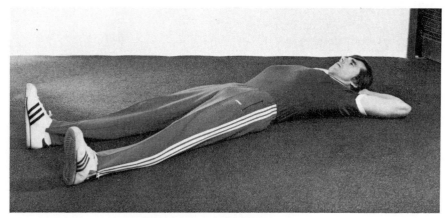

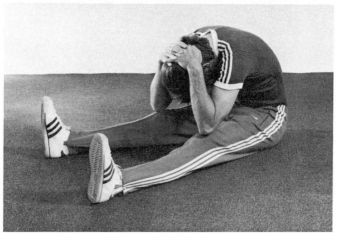

# EXERCISE 13   SIT-UPS WITH FOLDED ARMS

## Starting Position

Lie on back, legs together, arms folded across chest.

## Action

Raise body in rolling motion from waist and bend forward as far as possible. Lower body in rolling motion to original position. Repeat.

## Repetitions

Beginners    : None
Intermediate : 6 times
Advanced     : 8 times

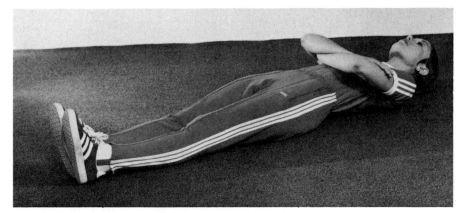

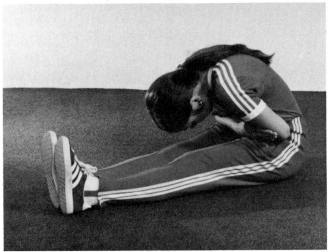

## EXERCISE 14 SIT-UP BENDING KNEES

### Starting Position

Lie on back, legs together, arms over head at full extension.
*Note:* Exercise may also be done with arms behind head or arms extended to sides.

### Action

Raise body in rolling motion from waist swinging arms over head and to front, bending knees to chest at same time. Lower upper and lower body at same time to original position. Repeat.

### Repetitions

Beginners     : 4 times
Intermediate : 6 times
Advanced     : 8 times

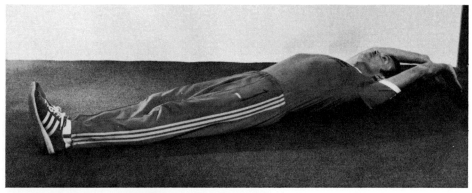

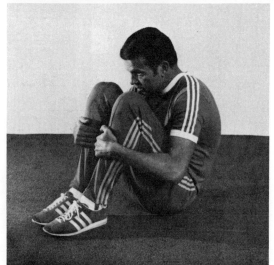

## EXERCISE 15　SIT-UP WITH BENT KNEES

### Starting Position

Lie on back, legs bent with feet as close to seat as possible. Hands behind head.

### Action

Raise body in rolling motion from waist until you are in a sitting position. Try to keep legs bent as tightly as possible and feet on floor. Lower upper body to original position. Repeat sequence.

### Repetitions

Beginners　　 : None
Intermediate : None
Advanced　　 : sets of 8

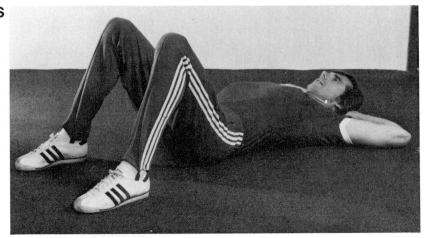

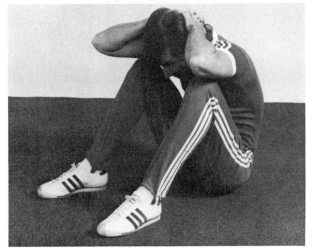

# EXERCISE 16   QUARTER SIT-UP AND HOLD

## Starting Position

Lie on back, legs together flat on floor. Arms at sides.

*Note:* Exercise can also be done with legs slightly bent, feet flat on floor.

## Action

Raise body in rolling motion from waist until body is at no more than 45 degree angle. Arms extended in front of body. Hold position for a count of 4 or 8 then lower to original position. Repeat.

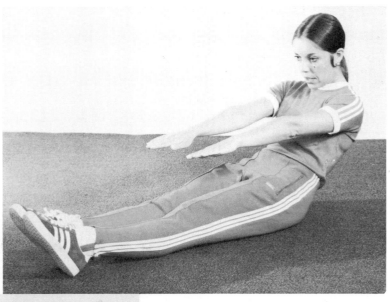

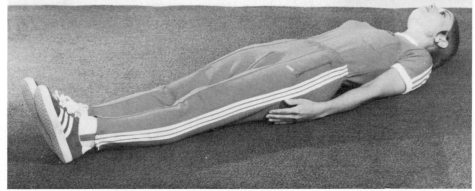

## Repetitions

Beginners      : None
Intermediate : 2 times
Advanced      : 4 times

# EXERCISE 17   V-SIT—FOUR COUNT

## Starting Position

Lie on back, legs together. Arms at sides.

*Note:* Exercise may also be done with hands behind head or across chest.

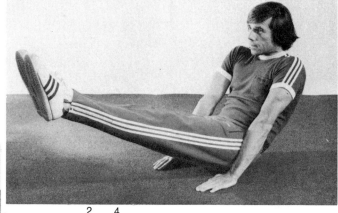

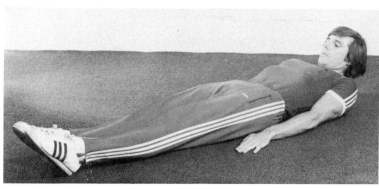

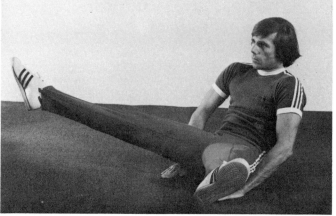

1
5

2   4

3

## Action

Raise upper and lower body at waist, rolling upper body until you are in a "V" position. Spread legs apart, bring legs together, lower body to original position. Repeat sequence.

## Repetitions

Beginners     : None
Intermediate : 2 times
Advanced     : 4 times

# EXERCISE 18   V-SIT WITH LEGS OFF GROUND

## Starting Position

Lie on back, legs apart and about 4 to 6 inches off ground. Arms at sides.

*Note:* Exercise may also be done with hands behind head or across chest.

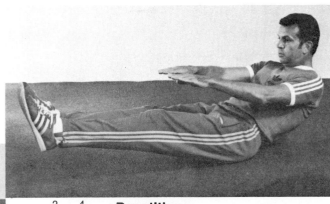

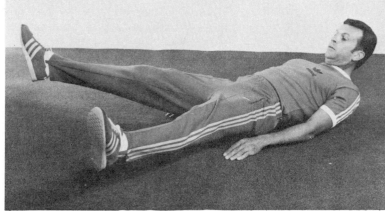

2    4

1

5

3

## Repetitions

Beginners      : None
Intermediate : None
Advanced      : Sets of 4–8

## Action

Raise upper and lower body bringing feet together, until you are in a "V" position. Spread legs apart, bring legs together, lower body to original position spreading legs apart and keeping them off floor. Repeat sequence.

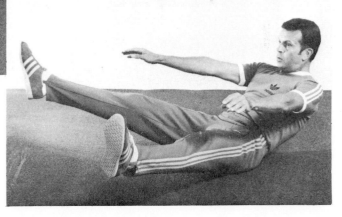

# EXERCISE 19  EXTENDED 3-ANGLE V-SIT

## Starting Position

Lie on back, legs together, hands at sides.

## Repetitions

Beginners     : None
Intermediate : None
Advanced     : 2–4 times

## Action

Raise upper and lower body 8 inches off floor. Hold for 2 counts. Raise upper and lower body another 8 inches off the floor. Hold for another 2 count. Raise upper and lower body to a tight "V" position, and grasp legs at thigh. Hold for 2 counts. Lower body in reverse sequence. Rest in original position for 2 counts and repeat exercise.

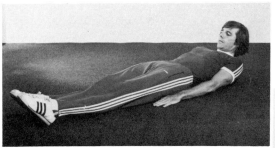

1

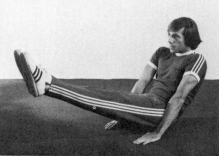

3

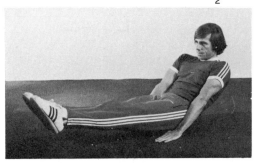

2

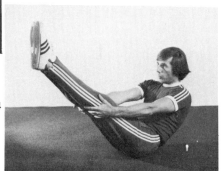

4

## EXERCISE 20   RAISED LEG SPREAD

### Starting Position

Lie on back, hands under seat, feet together, knees not bent, legs raised off ground 6 inches.

*Note:* Be sure head is bent up off floor to prevent back from being arched. Keep back flat on floor.

### Action

On first count spread legs apart. On second count bring legs back to original position. Repeat.

### Repetitions

Beginners    : 4 times
Intermediate : 6 times
Advanced     : 8–10 times

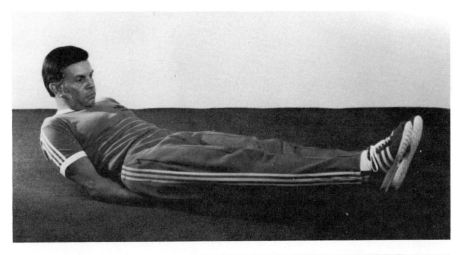

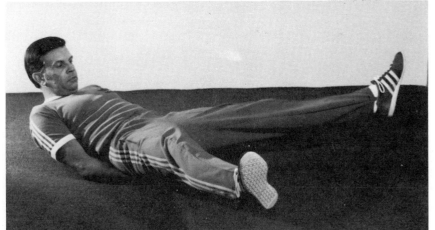

## EXERCISE 21   RAISED LEG CROSSOVER

### Starting Position

Lie on back, hands under seat, legs apart, knees not bent. Legs raised off ground 6 inches.

*Note:* Be sure head is bent up off floor to prevent back from arching. Keep back flat on floor.

### Action

With a swinging motion cross right leg over left. Swing apart and cross left over right. Repeat.

### Repetitions

Beginners    : 4 times
Intermediate : 6 times
Advanced    : 8–10 times

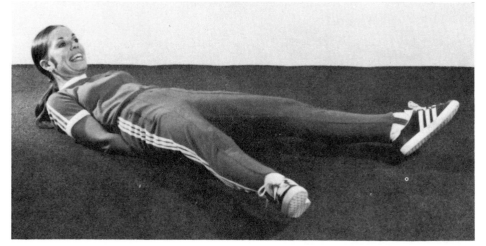

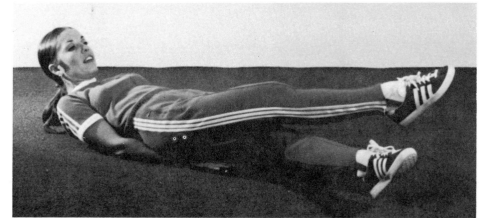

## EXERCISE 22   FLUTTER KICK AND SWAY

### Starting Position

Lie on back, hands under seat, feet together, knees not bent. Legs raised off ground 6 inches.

*Note:* Be sure head is bent up off floor to prevent back from arching. Keep back flat on floor.

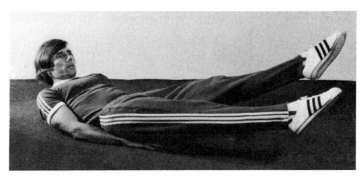

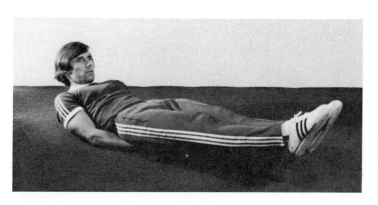

### Repetitions

Beginners     : None
Intermediate : 2 times side to side
Advanced     : 4–6 times side to side

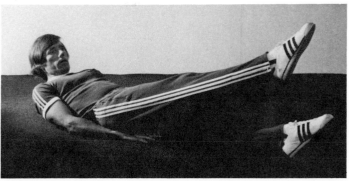

### Action

With a short kicking motion from hips *do not* bend knees, move legs up and down while swaying legs from right to left and back. Repeat.

## EXERCISE 23   CIRCLE LEG RAISE

### Starting Position

Lie on back, hands under seat, feet together, knees not bent. Legs raised off ground 6 inches.

*Note:* Be sure head is bent up off floor to prevent back from arching. Keep back flat on floor.

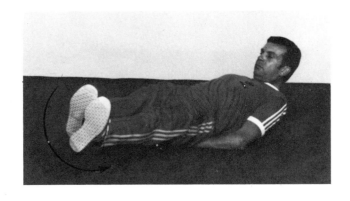

### Action

Rotate legs in a wide circular motion clockwise and then counterclockwise. Repeat.

### Repetitions

Beginners    : None
Intermediate : 3 times each way
Advanced     : 5–8 times each way

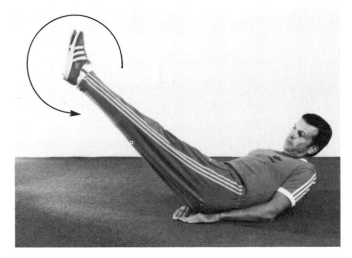

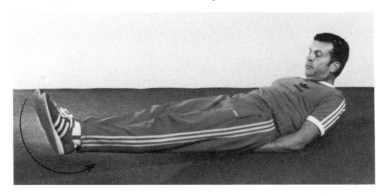

# EXERCISE 24   OVERHEAD LEG SPREAD

## Starting Position

Lie on back with legs up over head well forward. Arms to sides. You should be supported by head, neck, and shoulders.

## Action

Spread legs apart and together. Repeat.

## Repetitions

Beginners     : 6 times
Intermediate : 8 times
Advanced     : 8 times

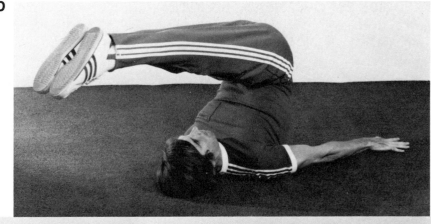

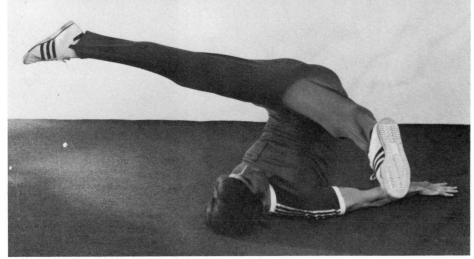

# EXERCISE 25   OVERHEAD LEG KICK

## Starting Position

Lie on back with legs up over head well forward. Arms to sides. You should be supported by head, neck, and shoulders.

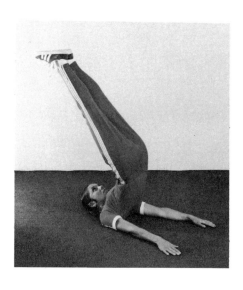

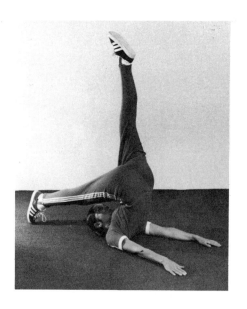

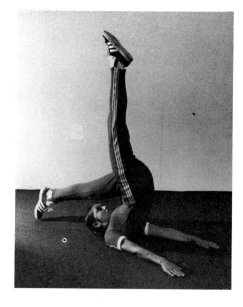

## Action

Kick legs down in front of head until they touch the floor, then raise and reverse. Repeat.

## Repetitions

Beginners    : None
Intermediate : 4–6 times
Advanced     : 8–10 times

# EXERCISE 26  BICYCLE KICK

## Starting Position

Lie on back with legs straight up, hands at waist for support. Raise up onto head, neck, and shoulders.

*Note:* It is permissible to extend arms to sides as shown in Exercise 25.

## Action

Kick right leg up and bend left leg down to chest. Reverse. Repeat in rapid succession.

## Repetitions

Beginners    : 10 times
Intermediate : 15 times
Advanced     : 20–25 times

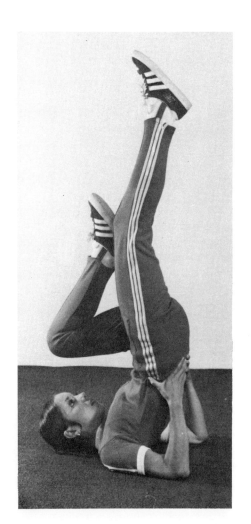
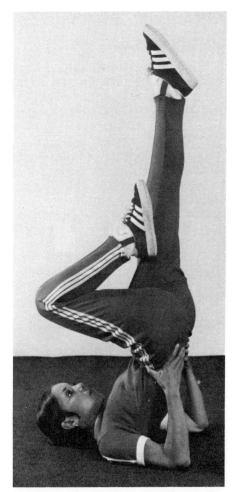

## EXERCISE 27   KNEES TO CHEST

### Starting Position

Sitting up on floor, extend arms slightly to sides and to rear, palms down flat on floor, legs straight out in front.

### Action

Raise legs slightly off floor and bend knees into chest, pulling in as close as possible. Straighten legs to original position. Repeat.

Note: Exercise can also be done by swinging arms in to grasp legs and squeeze.

Exercise can also be done with feet constantly about 6 inches off floor (Advanced only).

### Repetitions

Beginners    : 8 times
Intermediate : 8 times
Advanced    : 8 times

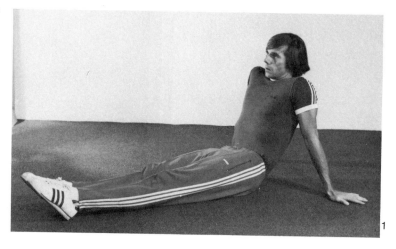

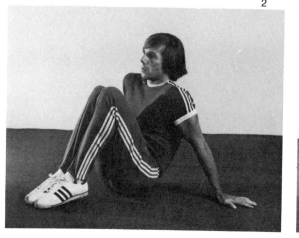

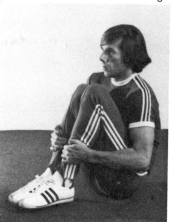

# EXERCISE 28　LEGS APART

## Starting Position

Sitting up on floor, extend arms slightly to sides and to the rear, palms down flat on floor, legs straight out front.

## Action

Spread legs apart and back together keeping knees as straight as possible. Repeat.

*Note:* Exercise can also be done with feet about 6 inches off floor (Advanced only).

## Repetitions

Beginners　　　 : 8 times
Intermediate : 8 times
Advanced　　　: 8 times

*Note:* Exercises 27 and 28 may also be combined—e.g., one exercise 27, one exercise 28, and repeat.

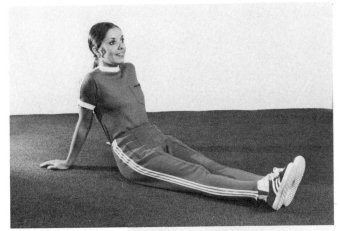

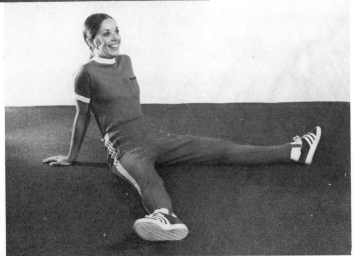

# EXERCISE 29   ROWING MOTION AND LEG SPREAD

## Starting Position

Sit on floor in V-sit position, legs 6 inches off floor, back raised in curved position, arms extended out front.

## Action

Spread arms and legs apart; return to original position on second movement. Pull hands and knees to chest on third movement. Return to original position and repeat sequence.

## Repetitions

Beginners    : None
Intermediate : None
Advanced     : 6–8 times

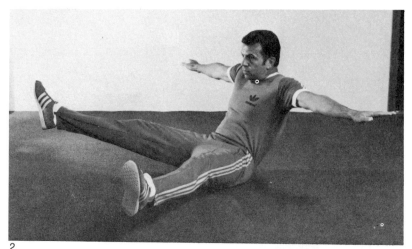

2

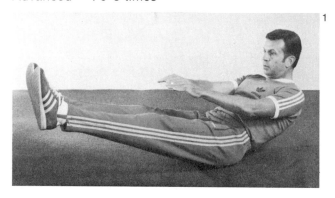

1

3

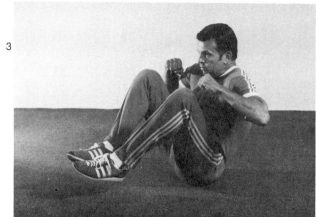

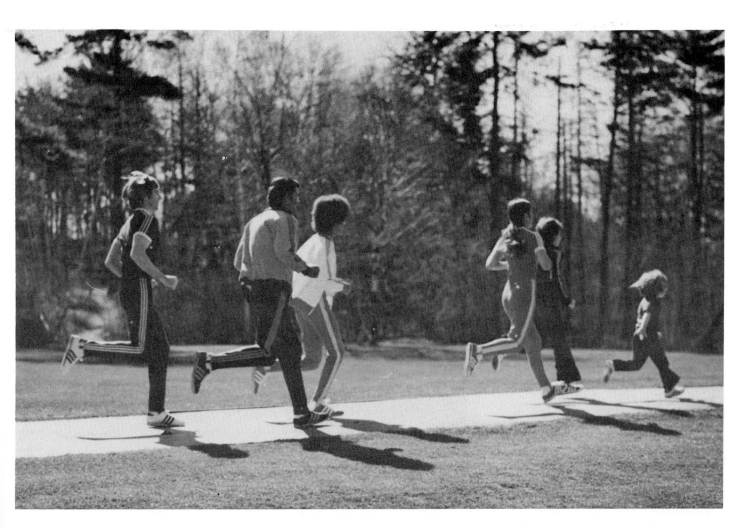

# The Cool-Down

This last portion of the program is one of the most essential.

After any exercise routine where you have substantially increased your pulse rate it is not wise to come to an abrupt conclusion.

The purpose of the cool-down is to return the body to its normal functioning level on a gradual basis.

The exercises in this portion are the same as those for the warm-up or the loosen-up, but are performed at a slower, more relaxed pace.

Specific exercises are now shown in this section. Therefore, when doing your program follow the exercises in the Warm-Up or Loosen-Up sections.

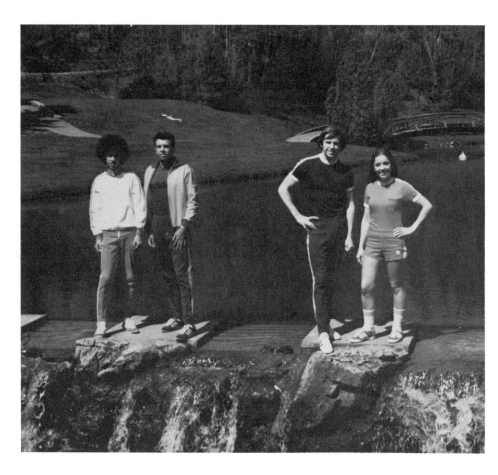

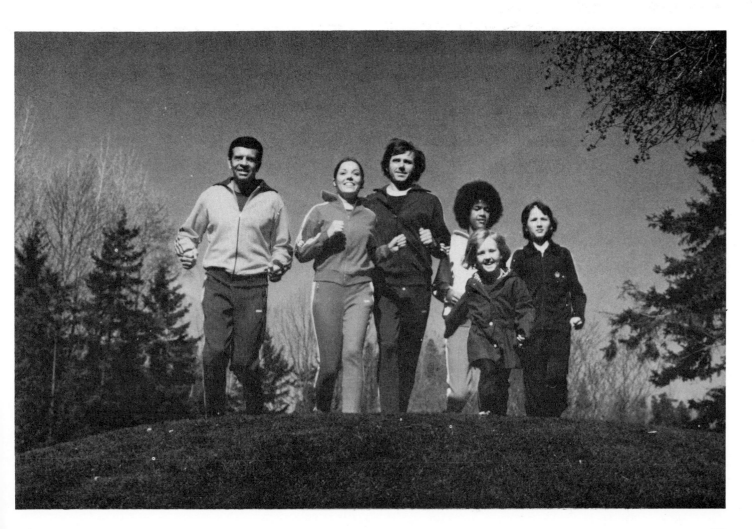

# Sample Programs For

## THE BEGINNER
## THE INTERMEDIATE
## THE ADVANCED

Note: These suggested programs can of course be varied and/or accelerated as your condition dictates. In the case of a group program, accelerate the intensity as the class progresses.

## THE BEGINNER PROGRAM

### Warm-Up

1. Run approx. ¼ mile: beginning with a slow jog gradually increasing pace.
2. Quick March
   - Arm Circles (Exercise 5)
   - Arm Rowing (Exercise 6)
   - Arm Side Extension (Exercise 7)
   - Overhead Arm Swing (Exercise 10)
3. Straddle Hopping (Exercises 12, 13, & 14): about 8 of each.
4. Running on the Spot (Exercise 1)

TIME: Approx. 6 minutes. (Take a 15 to 30 second break if necessary.)

### Loosen-Up

1. Short Side Bend (Exercises 1 & 2)
2. Body Twist—Arms Extended (Exercise 3)
3. Single Side Arm Pull (Exercise 5)
4. Double Side Arm Pull (Exercise 6)
5. Crossover Toe Touch (Exercise 7)
6. Double Toe Touch—Shoulder Pull (Exercise 9)
7. Sitting Crossover Toe Touch (Exercise 11)
8. Mid Torso Raise (Exercise 14)
9. Crossover Leg Stretch (Exercise 16)

TIME: Approx. 6 minutes. (Take a 15 to 30 second break if necessary.)

### Stretching, Bending, Pulling

1. Deep Side Bend (Exercise 1)
2. Ankle Grasp and Pull (Exercise 5)
3. Deep Stretch and Twist (Exercise 6)
4. Toe Touch—Arm Swing (Exercise 7)
5. Rotating Waist Bend (Exercise 10)

TIME: Approx. 5 minutes. (Take a 15 to 30 second break if necessary.)

## Muscle Toning

Note: We combine some stretching, bending, and pulling exercises in this section for break periods. Such exercises are indicated by an asterisk in front of them.

1. Waist Push-Up (Exercise 1)
2. *Single Side Leg Raise (Exercise 11) (Left Leg)
3. Waist Push-Up (Exercise 1)
4. *Single Side Leg Raise (Exercise 11) (Right Leg)
5. Half Push-Up (Exercise 2)
6. *Double, Side Leg Raise (Exercise 12) (Left Side)
7. Half Push-Up (Exercise 2)
8. *Double, Side Leg Raise (Exercise 12) (Right Side)
9. Full Push-Up (Exercise 3)
10. *Extended Arm Raise (Exercise 13)
11. Full Push-Up (Exercise 3)
12. *Extended Leg Raise (Exercise 14)
13. Sit-Up, Full Extension (Exercise 10)
14. Sit-Up, Leg Grasp (Exercise 11)
15. Sit-Up, Full Extension (Exercise 10)
16. Sit-Up, Leg Grasp (Exercise 11)

Note: Exercise 11 may be alternated with Exercises 12, 13, 14, 15, and 16 as you or your class progress.
TIME: Approx. 6 minutes. (Take a 15 to 30 second break if necessary.)

## Cool-Down

Note: Use the Warm-Up exercises but at a slow pace and with loose relaxed motions.

1. Arm Circles (Exercise 5): Let the arms bend a little and the shoulders go heavy.
2. Arm Rowing (Exercise 6): Motion should be as above.
3. Straddle Hop (Exercise 12): Motion as above but let the arms hang to sides and flop from the shoulders.
4. Jogging (Exercise 2): At a slow easy pace gradually slowing to a walk.
TIME: Approx. 4 minutes.
TOTAL TIME: Approx. 30 minutes.

## THE INTERMEDIATE PROGRAM

### Warm-Up

1. Straddle Hopping (Exercise 12)
2. Straddle Hop, Extend Arms Shoulder High (Exercise 13)
3. Straddle Hop, Arm & Leg Crossover (Exercise 15)
4. Run approx. ¼ Mile (Exercise 3): Begin slowly gradually increasing pace. (If exercising indoors run on the spot— Exercise 1)
5. Quick March
   - Arm Circles (Exercise 5)
   - Arm Rowing (Exercise 6)
   - Arm Side Extension (Exercise 7)
   - Alternate Forward Arm Thrust (Exercise 8)
   - Ankle Grasp (Exercise 11)
6. Side Running (Exercise 19)
7. Running Approx. ¼ Mile (Exercise 3) Medium Speed.

TIME: Approx. 7 minutes. Continue on with next section of program without a break.

### Loosen-Up

1. Short Side Bend (Exercise 1)
2. Body Twist—Arms Bent (Exercise 4)
3. Single, Side Arm Pull (Exercise 5)
4. Double, Side Arm Pull (Exercise 6)
5. Crossover Toe Touch (Exercise 7)
6. Short Knee Bend (Exercise 8)
7. Double Toe Touch—Overhead Arm Extension (Exercise 10)
8. Sitting, Crossover Toe Touch (Exercise 11)
9. Sitting, Double Toe Touch— Overhead Arm Extension (Exercise 12)
10. Mid Torso Raise (Exercise 14)
11. Crossover Leg Stretch (Exercise 16)

TIME: Approx. 8 minutes. Continue on with next portion of program without a break.

### Stretching, Bending, Pulling

1. Deep Side Bends (Exercise 1)
2. Alternate Leg Burpees (Exercise 4)
3. Deep Stretch and Twist Left and Right (Exercise 6)
4. Toe Touch—Arm Swing (Exercise 7)
5. Alternate Toe Touch—Overhead Arm Extension (Exercise 8)
6. Rotating Waist Bend (Exercise 10)

TIME: Approx. 6 minutes. (Take a 10 second break if desired.)

### Muscle Toning

Note: We combine some stretching, bending and pulling exercises in this section for break periods. Such exercises are indicated by an asterisk in front of them.

1. Waist Push-Up (Exercise 1)
2. Full Push-Up (Exercise 3)
3. *Single Side Leg Raise Right (Exercise 11)
4. Full Push-Up (Exercise 3)
5. *Single Side Leg Raise Left (Exercise 11)
6. Half Push-Up (Exercise 2)

7. *Extended Arm Raise (Exercise 13)
8. Side Push-Up Right (Exercise 8)
9. Side Push-Up Left (Exercise 8)
10. Sit-Up Full Extension (Exercise 10)
11. Sit-Up with Leg Grasp (Exercise 11)
12. Sit-Up, Full Extension (Exercise 10)
13. Sit-Up, Hands Behind Head (Exercise 12)
14. V-Sit, Four Count (Exercise 17)
15. Sit-Up Full Extension (Exercise 10)
16. Quarter Sit-Up and Hold Count of 4 (Exercise 16)
17. Raised Leg Spread (Exercise 20)
18. Overhead Leg Spread (Exercise 24)
19. Knees to Chest (Exercise 27)
20. Legs Apart (Exercise 28)
TIME: Approx. 8 minutes. (Continue on with next portion of program without a break.)

## Cool-Down

Note: Use the Loosen-Up Exercises but at a slow pace and with loose relaxed motions.
1. Short Side Bend (Exercise 1)
2. Body Twist—Arms Extended (Exercise 3): Let the arms go limp and the shoulders heavy.
3. Crossover Toe Touch (Exercise 7): Let the body sway from side to side and don't raise up to return to original position each time.
4. Double Toe Touch—Overhead Arm Extension (Exercise 10): Let the body fall forward and let the elbows bend when they are raised over the head.
5. Hopping on the spot. Use a number of variations but in an easy relaxed motion.
TIME: Approx. 4 minutes.
TOTAL TIME: Approx. 33—35 minutes.

## THE ADVANCED PROGRAM

Note: This suggested format can of course be varied. When you can complete a program such as this in the time frame specified you should be in reasonably good overall condition. In the case of individuals or groups the exercises can and should be varied.

### Warm-Up

1. Straddle Hop (Exercise 12)
2. Straddle Hop, Extend Arms Shoulder High (Exercise 13)
3. Straddle Hop, Arm & Leg Crossover (Exercise 15)
4. Front-Back Stride Hop (Exercise 17)
5. Front-Back Stride Hop with Arm Raise (Exercise 18)
6. Forward Motion Side to Side Hop (Exercise 16)
7. Hopping Torso Twist (Exercise 22)
8. Straddle Hop (Exercise 12)
9. Running (Exercise 3)

10. Quick March
    - Arm Circles (Exercise 5)
    - Arm Rowing (Exercise 6)
    - Marching Body Twist (Exercise 9)
    - Overhead Arm Swing (Exercise 10)
11. Side Running (Exercise 19)
12. Side Running—Arm Swing (Exercise 20)
13. Quick March—Arm Side Extension (Exercise 7)
14. Running (Exercise 3)

TIME: Approx. 12 minutes. (Continue on with next section without a break.)

## Loosen-Up

1. Short Side Bend (Exercise 1)
2. Short Side Bend with Arm Raise (Exercise 2)
3. Body Twist—Arms Bent (Exercise 4)
4. Single Side Arm Pull (Exercise 5)
5. Double Side Arm Pull (Exercise 6)
6. Crossover Toe Touch (Exercise 7)
7. Double Toe Touch—Overhead Arm Extension (Exercise 10)
8. Sitting Crossover Toe Touch (Exercise 11)
9. Mid Torso Raise (Exercise 14)
10. Extended Leg Raise (Exercise 15)
11. Crossover Leg Stretch (Exercise 16)

TIME: Approx. 5 minutes. (Continue on with next section without a break.)

Note: There are more exercises in a shorter period of time here but the pace should be accelerated.

## Stretching, Bending, Pulling

1. Deep Side Bend (Exercise 1)
2. Deep Stretch and Twist (Exercise 6) (left and right)
3. Toe Touch—Arm Swing (Exercise 7)
4. Alternate Toe Touch—Overhead Arm Extension (Exercise 8)
5. Alternate Leg Burpees (Exercise 4)
6. Rotating Waist Bend (Exercise 10)

TIME: Approx. 4–5 minutes. (Continue on with next section without a break.)

Note: In the Advanced Program we usually have a fast run or slow run with sprints at this point. See Warm-Up Exercise 4.

TIME: Approx. 3 minutes.

## Muscle Toning

Note: We combine some stretching, bending and pulling exercises in this section for break periods. Such exercises are indicated by an asterisk.
1. Full Push-Up (Exercise 3)
2. *Single Side Leg Raise Left Leg (Exercise 11)
3. Full Push-Up (Exercise 3)
4. *Single Side Leg Raise Right Leg (Exercise 11)
5. Full Push-Up (Exercise 3)
6. *Double Side Leg Raise Left Side (Exercise 12)
7. Full Push-Up (Exercise 3)
8. *Double Side Leg Raise Right Side (Exercise 12)
9. Full Push-Up (Exercise 3)
10. *Extended Arm Raise (Exercise 13)
11. Push-Up—Four Count (Exercise 5)
12. *Extended Leg Raise (Exercise 14)
13. Side Push-Up, Left Side (Exercise 8)
14. Side Push-Up, Right Side (Exercise 8)
15. *Torso Bends (Exercise 17)
16. Waist Push-Up (Exercise 1)
17. Sit-Up Full Extension (Exercise 10)
18. Sit-Up With Leg Grasp (Exercise 11)
19. V-Sit—Four Count (Exercise 17)
20. Sit-Up Full Extension (Exercise 10)
21. Sit-Up—Hands Behind Head (Exercise 12)
22. Extended Triangled V-Sit (Exercise 19)
23. Raised Leg Spread (Exercise 20)
24. Raised Leg Crossover (Exercise 21)
25. Overhead Leg Spread (Exercise 24)
26. Overhead Leg Kick (Exercise 25)
27. Flutter Kick and Sway (Exercise 22)
28. Knees to Chest (Exercise 27)
29. Legs Apart (Exercise 28)
TIME: Approx. 10 minutes. (Continue on with next section without a break.)

## Cool-Down

Note: Use the Loosen-Up exercises but at a slow pace and with loose relaxed motions.
1. Short Side Bend (Exercise 1)
2. Short Side Bend With Arm Raise (Exercise 2)
3. Body Twist—Arms Extended (Exercise 3): Let the arms go limp and the shoulders heavy.
4. Double Toe Touch—Overhead Arm Extension (Exercise 10): Let the body fall forward and let the elbows bend when they are raised over the head.
5. Crossover Toe Touch (Exercise 7): Let the body sway from side to side and don't raise up to return to original position each time.
6. Hopping on the spot. Use a number of variations but in an easy relaxed motion.
TIME: Approx. 4–5 minutes.
TOTAL TIME: Approx. 40 minutes.

# Speciality Exercises

This group of exercises is used after the basic exercise program has been completed, but before the cool-down.

It can be detrimental to do these exercises before you have gone through a regular conditioning routine, because some of these exercises do strain specific muscle groups.

Execute the exercises as explained and avoid excessive speed. As in all other exercises speed is not as important as getting into the exercise.

These exercises are separated by type.

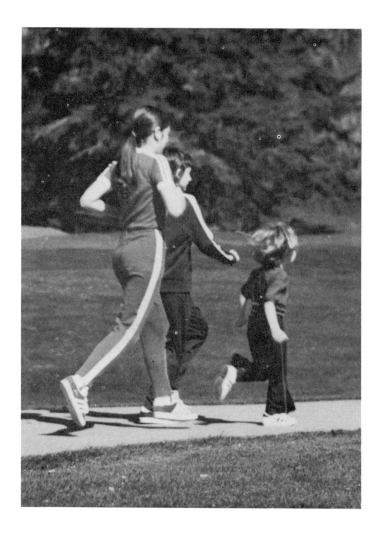

# EXERCISE 1   STRIDE JUMP WITH VARIABLE ARM RAISE

## Purpose: Co-ordination

## Starting Position

Stand erect, feet together, arms to sides.

## Action

On first movement spread legs apart, at same time raising right arm to the side shoulder high and raise left arm to the front up over the head. On second movement return legs and arms to original position. On third movement raise left arm to the side shoulder high and right arm to the front up over the head. On fourth movement return to original position. Repeat sequence 15 to 20 times.

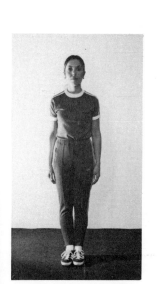
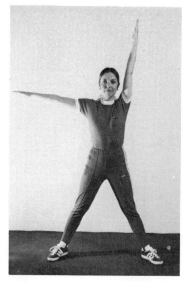
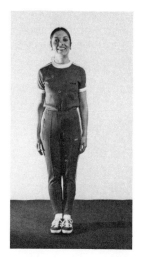
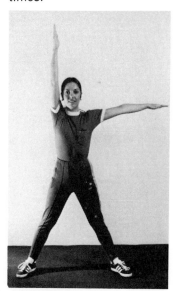

# EXERCISE 2   DOUBLE STRIDE JUMP WITH ARM RAISE

## Purpose: Co-ordination

### Starting Position

Stand erect, feet together, arms to sides.

### Action

On first movement spread legs apart and raise both arms to sides up over the head. On second movement lower arms to sides and hop keeping legs apart. On third movement raise arms to sides up over the head and bring legs together. On fourth movement lower arms to sides and hop keeping legs together. Repeat sequence 15 to 20 times.

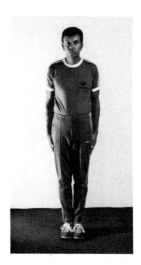
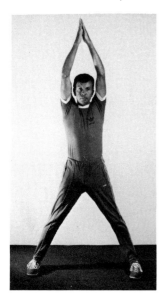
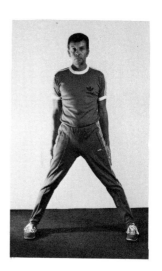
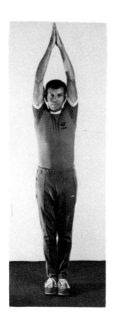

# EXERCISE 3  STRIDE JUMP WITH FORWARD/BACKWARD ARM SWING

## Purpose: Co-ordination

### Starting Position

Stand erect, feet together, arms to sides.

### Action

On first movement spread legs apart and raise right arm shoulder high to the front and left arm shoulder high to the rear. On second movement bring legs together and swing right arm to the rear and left arm to the front. Repeat sequence 15 to 20 times.

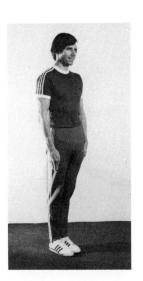
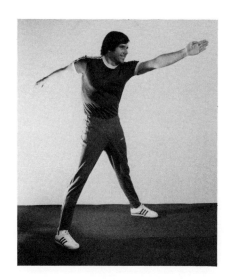
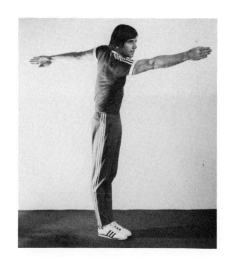

# EXERCISE 4  STEP UPS

## Purpose: Strengthen knees and legs

## Starting Position

*Note:* Use the bottom step or a low
bench or box.
Stand erect, arms at sides, straight
down or bent at elbows.

## Action

Step up with right leg followed by
left. Step down with right leg followed by left. Repeat sequence 20
times. Rest 10 seconds, then reverse
with left leg followed by right.

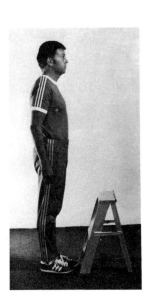

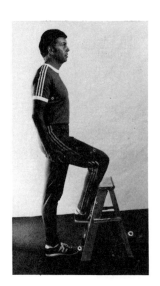

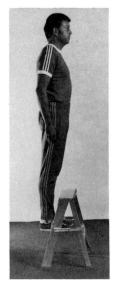

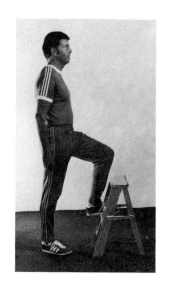

# EXERCISE 5  SINGLE LEG BODY LIFT

## Purpose: 1. Strengthen knees and legs
##               2. Balance

### Starting Position

*Note:* Use the bottom step or a low
bench or box.
Stand erect, arms at sides. Place left
foot on box.

### Action

Lift body with left leg by straightening leg. *Do not* rest right leg on
step. Lower body slowly by bending
left leg.
*Note:* Try not to use hands to
balance.
Repeat sequence 15 times,
then reverse to right leg.

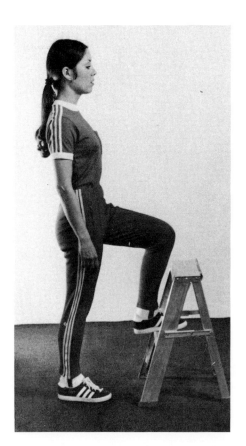
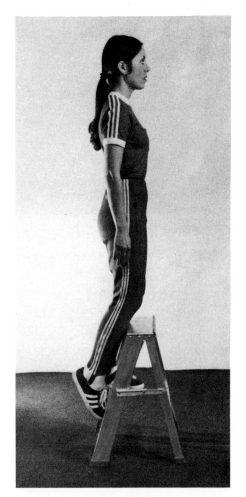

## EXERCISE 6  BENCH STRADDLE JUMP (MOVING)

**Purpose: 1. Strengthen legs**
**2. Balance**
**3. Agility**

### Starting Position

*Note:* For this exercise you will require a long low bench 8 to 10 inches wide.

Stand on bench, feet together, hands on hips.

### Action

Moving forward, jump down from bench, one foot on each side. Let knees bend slightly then spring back up on bench to original position, but moving forward. Repeat sequence 15 times and increase to between 30 and 40 as you can.

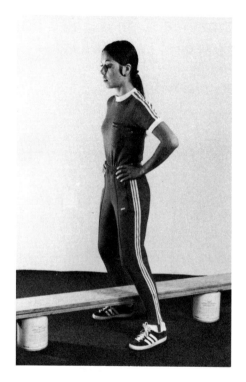
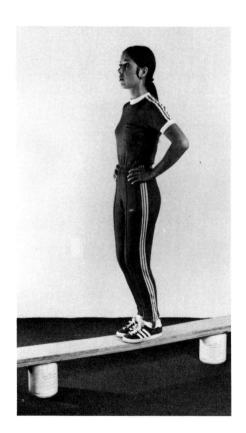

## EXERCISE 7   BENCH SIDE TO SIDE JUMP

**Purpose: 1. Strengthen legs**
**2. Balance**
**3. Agility**

### Starting Position

*Note:* For this exercise you will require a long low bench 8 to 10 inches wide.

Stand at one side of bench, about 6 to 8 inches from bench, feet together with hands on hips.

### Action

Lean slightly to opposite side of bench, spring off floor, keeping feet together and land on opposite side of bench. Then return to original side in same manner. *Do Not Spread Feet Apart.* Move forward with each jump. Repeat sequence 15 times and increase to between 30 and 40 as you can.

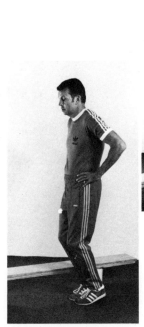
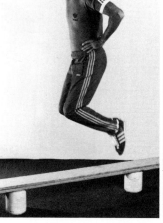
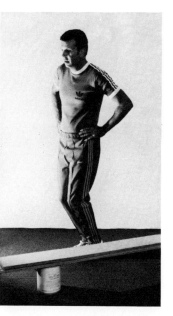

# EXERCISE 8 WALKING ON TOES

## Purpose: Strengthen lower legs and ankles

### Starting Position

Stand erect, hands on hips and raise up on toes.

### Action

Take regular walking stride and keep feet bent in original toe position. Do *not* bend knees. Walk at least 20 to 30 steps.

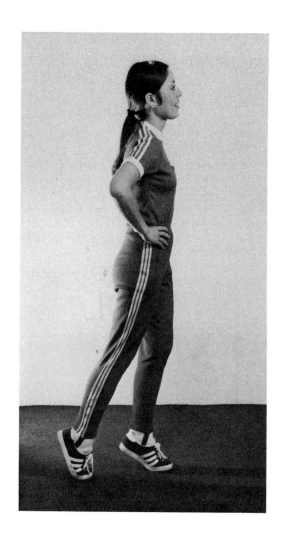

# EXERCISE 9   WALKING ON HEELS

## Purpose: Stretch leg muscles and tendons

### Starting Position

Stand erect, hands on hips and raise toes up until you are balancing on heels.

### Action

Take regular walking stride and remain on heels. Do *not* bend knees. Walk at least 20 to 30 steps.

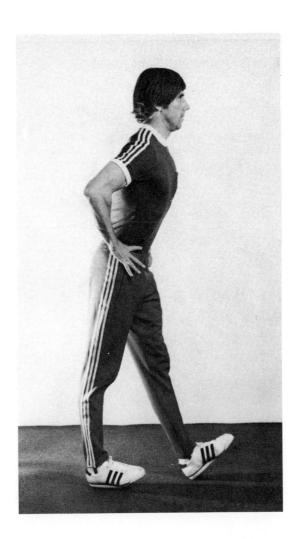

# EXERCISE 10   DOUBLE ANKLE/CALF PULL

## Purpose: Strengthen ankles and lower legs

### Starting Position

Place hands slightly above head, arms fully extended, palms on wall. Keeping hands on wall step back as far as you can until only your toes are on the ground. Keep knees straight.

### Action

Lower heels to the floor slowly, keeping hands on wall. Raise up slowly as far as you can. Repeat sequence at least 10 times.

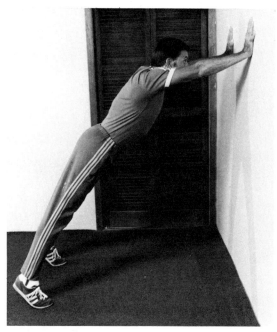 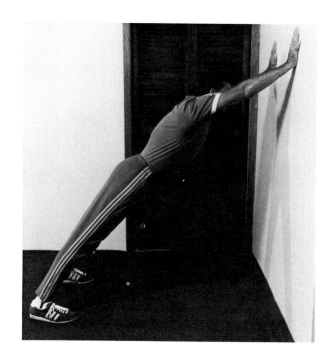

# EXERCISE 11   CLOSED EYED DIVERS STANCE

## Purpose: Balance

## Starting Position

Stand on toes. Toes 6 inches apart, heels together. Arms extended in front of you shoulder high. Do not let hands touch.

## Action

Close your eyes. Have someone time you and remain in position for 1 minute. Repeat exercise as required until you can remain steady for 1 minute.

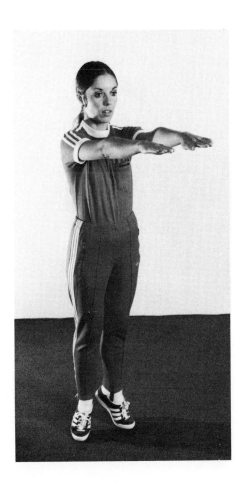
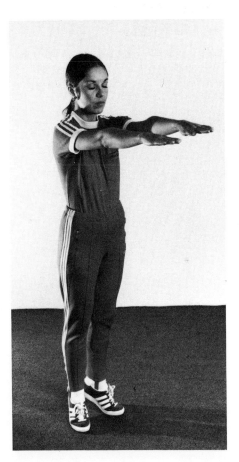

# EXERCISE 12   CIRCLE ROTATE

## Purpose: Balance

## Starting Position

Place your finger on floor (left or right index). Keep head down and remain in a crouched walking position.

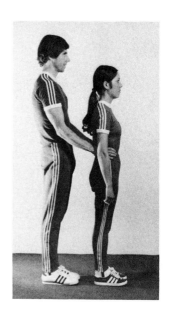

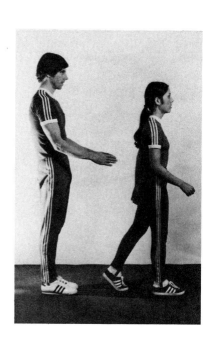

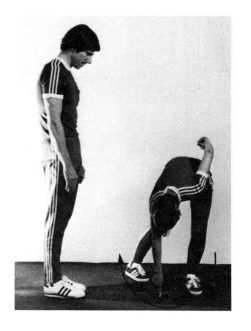

## Action

Walk in a circle around your finger 10 times in 30 seconds. Stand up (someone may steady you for 5 seconds) then walk a straight line for 10 feet. Repeat as required.

# EXERCISE 13  HAMSTRING STRETCH

## Purpose: Strengthen hamstrings

## Starting Position

Facing a wall, place heel against wall, toe up. Keep leg straight. Other leg should be bent.

## Action

Raise leg, with heel against wall slightly by straightening opposite leg. Then relax keeping heel against wall. *Caution:* Do not attempt this exercise unless you are well warmed up. Repeat 5 times and then reverse to other leg.

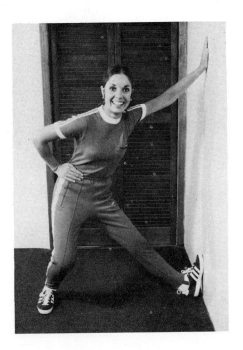
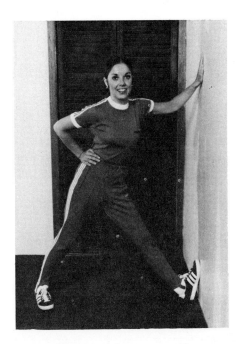

## EXERCISE 14    CHIN UPS

### Purpose: Strengthen upper arms and shoulders

### Starting Position

*Note:* For this exercise you will need a cross bar that will support your weight. Bar should be slightly higher than you will be with your arms fully extended over your head.

Grasp bar with your palms facing you.

### Action

Pull up until your chin is above bar, then lower yourself slowly until your arms are almost fully extended. Feet should not touch the ground. Repeat 6 to 8 times.

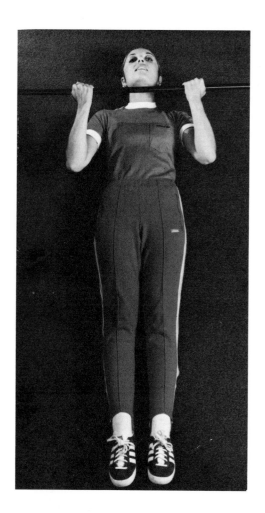

# EXERCISE 15   CRAB WALK

## Purpose: Agility

## Starting Position

*Note:* For this exercise you need a leader who will give orders and therefore your head should remain up.

Place hands and feet on floor with knees bent but not touching floor.

## Action

As leader points to indicate your direction you are to move there as quickly as possible. Keep watching leader for signals to change direction. Follow leader's instructions for three 20 second intervals, each one separated by a 15 second rest period.

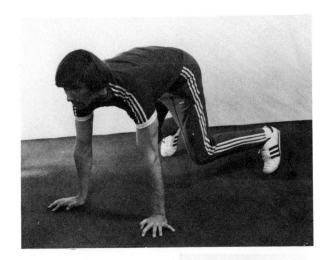

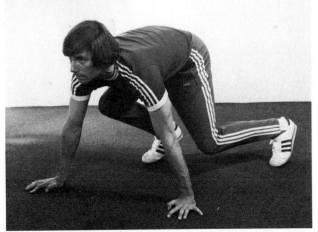

# EXERCISE 16   ZIG-ZAG RUN

**Purpose: Agility**

**Starting Position**

*Note:* For this exercise you will need 5 objects (chairs, boxes, poles, etc.). Place about 4 feet apart in a line.

Stand erect behind first object facing it.

Direction of Running

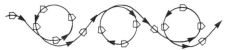

*Note:* At all times face forward.

2. Move between first and second chair. Remember to always face forward.

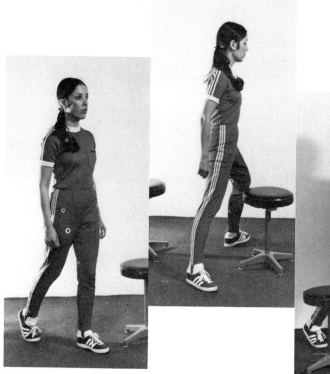

**Action**

1. Pass around right side of first chair.

3. Move back around first chair and keep facing forward.

4. Continue to move around first chair and then move between first and second chair.

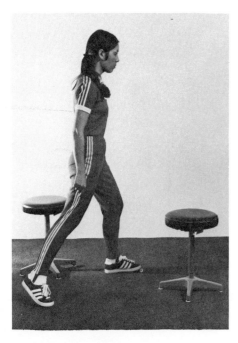

5. Move around left side of second chair.

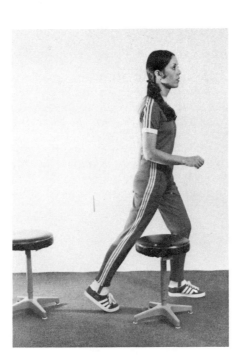

6. Move back around right hand side of second chair. Remember you must always face forward.

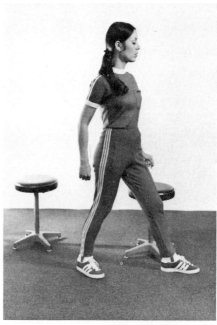

7. Move around second chair, going between second and third chair and continue in this sequence through all five chairs.

Rest 15 seconds and repeat.

# EXERCISE 17 HOP STEP AND JUMP

## Purpose: Agility

### Starting Position

*Note:* You must mark off about a 20 to 25 foot interval on the floor.

Stand about 5 to 6 feet behind the starting line. A long run is not necessary nor is it necessary to be at full speed when approaching the line.

### Action

Approach the start line at about one-half speed. Spring from the starting line with either foot. You must land in the jump area on the same foot you started on. This is the HOP. Then, moving forward STEP to the opposite foot and from this foot JUMP to the finish line. You should land outside the finish line. Repeat 3 to 5 times.

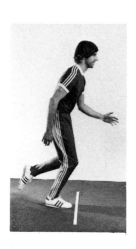
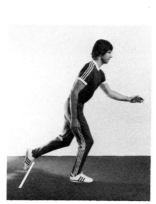
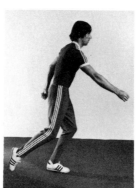
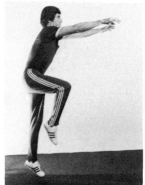
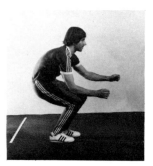

# EXERCISE 18   STANDING BROAD JUMP

## Purpose: Power

## Starting Position

*Note:* Mark off a starting point and a finishing point. The finishing point should be at least your height plus 1 foot.
Assume a slightly crouched position with your arms back.

## Action

Throwing your arms forward, jump as far as you can, landing in a squat position. Your heels must be past your finish line and you are not allowed to fall back. Repeat 2 to 3 times. Try to add a few more inches to your distance each time.

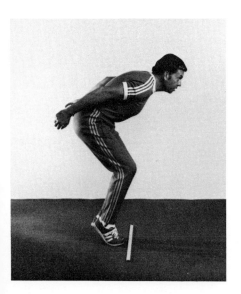

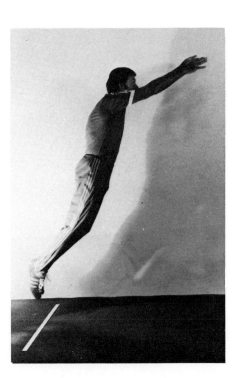

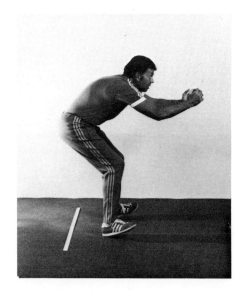

# EXERCISE 19   INWARD ANKLE BEND

## Purpose: Strengthen ankles

## Starting Position

Stand erect with feet bent in until you are resting on outer edge of foot.

## Action

Commence normal walking, keeping feet bent in. Take at least 15 to 20 steps.

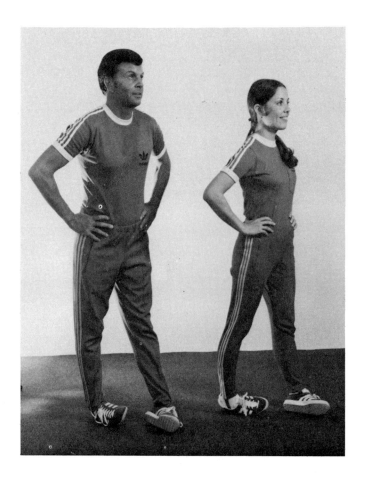

# EXERCISE 20   OUTWARD ANKLE BEND

## Purpose: Strengthen ankles

## Starting Position

Stand in a slightly squatted position with knees slightly bent bending feet outward until you are on inner edge of foot.

## Action

Commence walking, keeping feet bent outward. Take at least 15 to 20 steps.

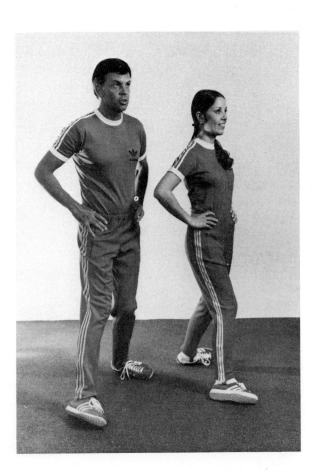

## EXERCISE 21   ANKLE ROTATE

### Purpose: Strengthen ankles

### Starting Position

Lie on back or sit in chair. Keep legs straight.

*Note:* This exercise can be done with no shoes on or it can be done with heavy shoes on to increase stress.

### Action

Slowly and deliberately rotate ankles to the right and then to the left. Rotate right 15 to 20 times and then reverse.

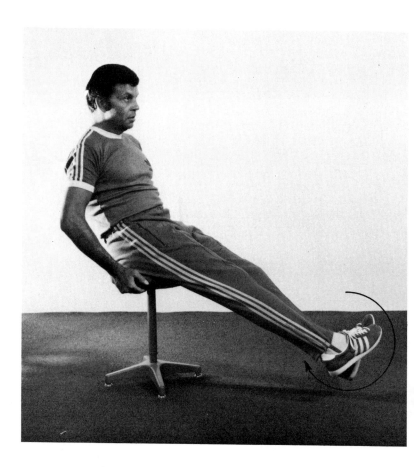

# EXERCISE 22 WRIST ROTATE

## Purpose: Strengthen wrists

## Starting Position

Extend arms to front or sides. Do not bend elbows.

*Note:* This exercise can be done with no additional weight or it can be done with any object grasped in hands to add weight and therefore additional stress.

## Action

Slowly and deliberately rotate wrists to the right and then to the left. Rotate right 15 to 20 times and then reverse.

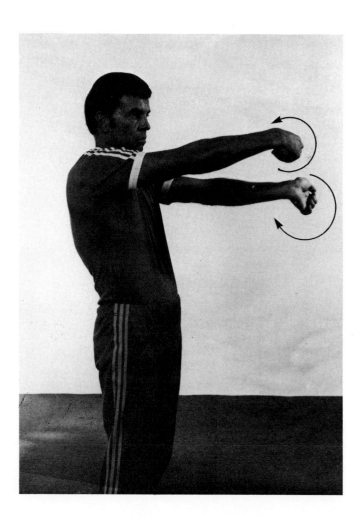

# EXERCISE 23   WRIST CURL

## Purpose: Strengthen wrists

## Starting Position

*Note:* Secure any weight (the heavier, the more stress involved) to a piece of cord at one end of cord and secure other end of cord to a dole or any object onto which it can be rolled. Cord with object attached should be about 1 foot shorter than distance from your shoulder to the floor.

Extend arms to front shoulder high and do not bend elbows. Grasp dole in both hands with heavy object fully extended.

## Action

Slowly roll cord onto dole using only a deliberate wrist action. When fully rolled up, slowly unroll cord until object is once again fully extended. Repeat sequence 5 or more times.

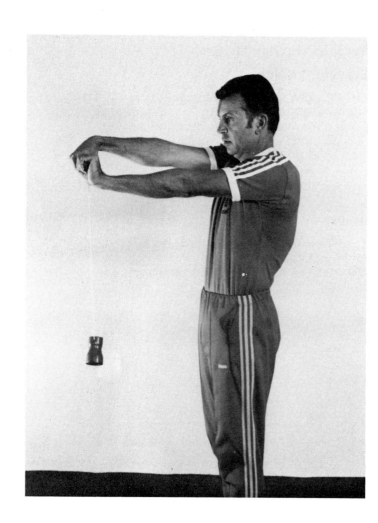

# EXERCISE 24  JACK SPRING

## Purpose: Agilty and Balance

## Starting Position

Stand erect, feet slightly apart, hands on hips.

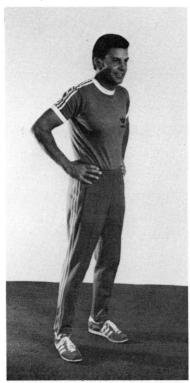

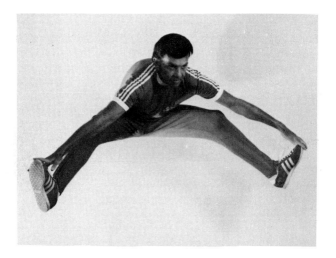

## Action

Jack spring from the standing position kicking legs out and bending body forward. Reach out with arms and touch toes when legs are waist high. Return to original position without losing balance. Repeat in rapid succession at least 5 times.

# Isometric Exercises

This method of exercising supplements daily activity.

It is designed to strengthen muscles to a degree attained previously only by a weight training program or other strenuous activity.

These exercises are used to develop strength and *should not* be considered a conditioning program.

They do not require special equipment and they can be done in a relatively short period of time.

Isometric exercises pit one set of muscles against another to achieve the desired result.

*Caution:* Some persons have claimed isometric exercises to be potentially harmful. Unlike most exercises outlined in my basic exercise programs, these exercises do put excess pressure on your system over and above that caused by your body weight.

I suggest that, for the first week at least, only about 40 to 50 per cent maximum exertion should be applied in the push and pull positions, gradually building up thereafter.

Do each exercise for no more than 6 seconds and hold your breath while doing each one. Relax completely for a few seconds after each exertion.

For maximum benefit, these exercises must be done every day and although one repetition of each exercise should result in increased strength for most people; 3 to 6 of each will improve your muscular endurance and strength.

It is claimed that you may as much as double your strength in only 20 weeks if you rigidly adhere to this program. The average increase appears to be between 3 and 5 per cent per week, however. Increases in strength depend on the person and the degree to which pressure is applied.

## EXERCISE 1   ARM CURL

### Purpose: Strengthen upper arms

### Starting Position

Stand or sit straight, elbows bent forearm parallel to floor, elbows against sides, palms up.

### Action

If standing, use low bar in gym. If seated, use heavy desk or table. Lift up as hard as possible, keeping elbows in.

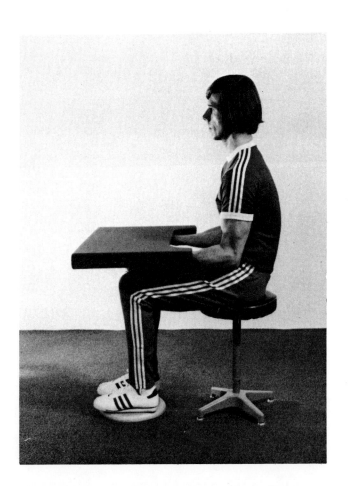

## EXERCISE 2   FORWARD ARM RAISE

### Purpose: Strengthen shoulder muscles

### Starting Position

Extend hands in front of body parallel to floor. Keep elbows straight.

### Action

If standing, use low bar in gym. If seated, use heavy desk or table. Lift up as hard as possible, keeping elbows straight.

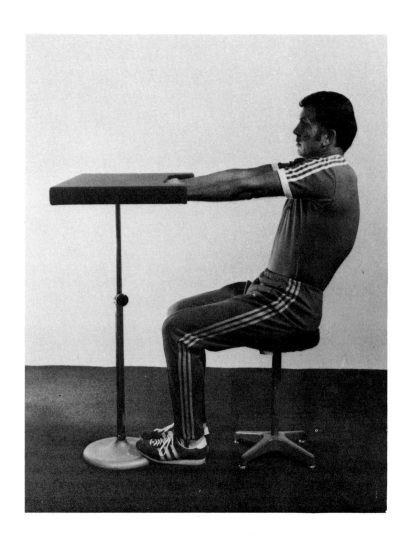

# EXERCISE 3   THE LATERAL RAISE

## Purpose: Strengthen shoulder muscles

## Starting Position

Stand straight in doorway, back of hands against sides of doorway.

## Action

Try to push arms out as hard as possible, keeping arms straight.

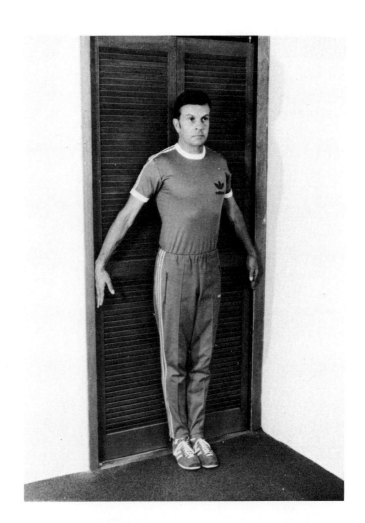

# EXERCISE 4   HAND PRESS

## Purpose: Strengthen upper arms (triceps), chest, and shoulders.

### Starting Position

Sit straight with chest out and arms across chest. Place one fist inside the other.

### Action

Push hands together as hard as possible using strength of arms and shoulders.

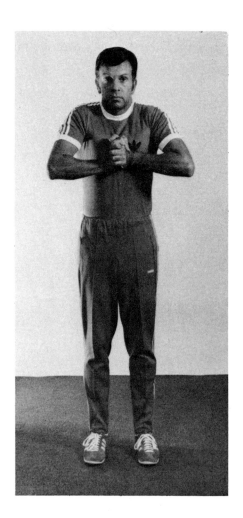

# EXERCISE 5   PULL UP

## Purpose: Strengthen arms and shoulders.

## Starting Position

Sit straight in chair. Grasp side of chair tightly with both hands.

## Action

Pull up as hard as possible.

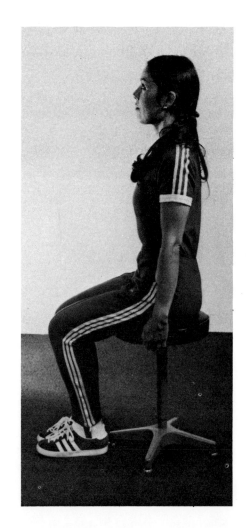

## EXERCISE 6   BODY LIFT

### Purpose: Strengthen shoulders, arms, and abdomen.

### Starting Position

Sitting straight in a chair, grasp sides of chair. Hold legs straight out.

### Action

Press down with hands and arms and attempt to lift body about 1 inch off the chair.

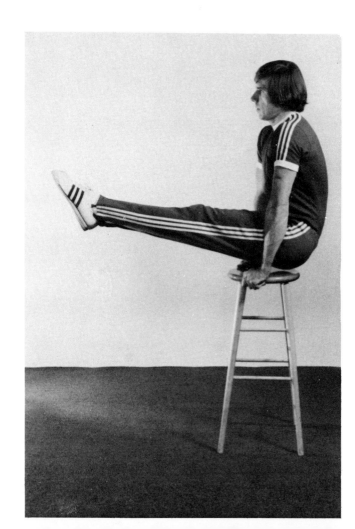

# EXERCISE 7  TUMMY TIGHTENER

## Purpose: Strengthen abdominal muscles and waist

### Starting Position

Sit with legs straight out. Bend forward and grasp legs midway between ankle and knee.

### Action

Press down with the hands and
press up against hands with the
legs.

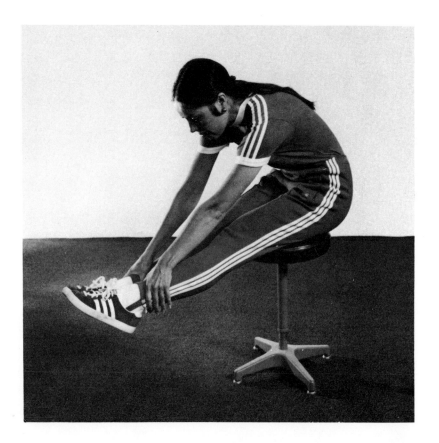

## EXERCISE 8   NECK PRESS

### Purpose: Strengthen the neck

### Starting Position

Sitting straight in chair, clasp hands behind neck. Bend elbows forward.

### Action

Pull forward with hands and simultaneously press the head back.

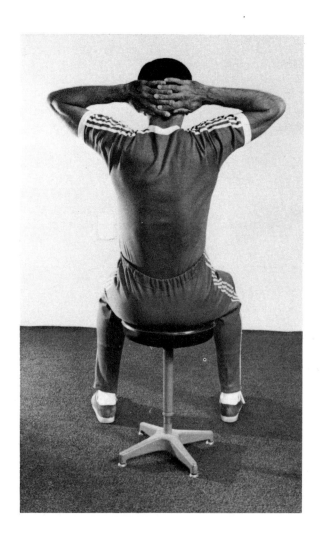

# EXERCISE 9 BACK PULL

## Purpose: Strengthen the back

## Starting Position

Sitting straight, keeping back as straight as possible lean forward until you can grasp your legs.

## Action

Pull straight up using back muscles only.

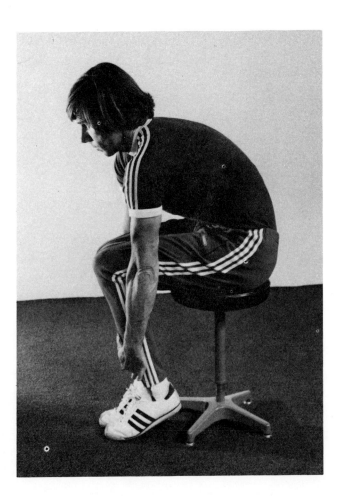

## EXERCISE 10   CROSSOVER

### Purpose: Strengthen chest and legs

### Starting Position

Sitting straight, place feet about 6 inches apart, lean forward and place hands against inside of opposite knees.

### Action

Press knees together as hard as possible while trying to hold them apart with hands.

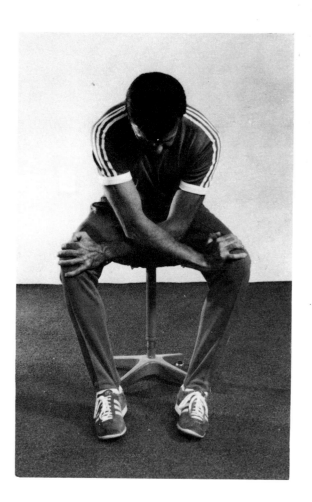

# EXERCISE 11   LEG SQUEEZER

## Purpose: Strengthen legs and ankles

### Starting Position

Sit on stool or edge of chair, lean back and hold legs straight out. Hook one foot over the other and hold tightly.

### Action

Attempt to pull feet apart.

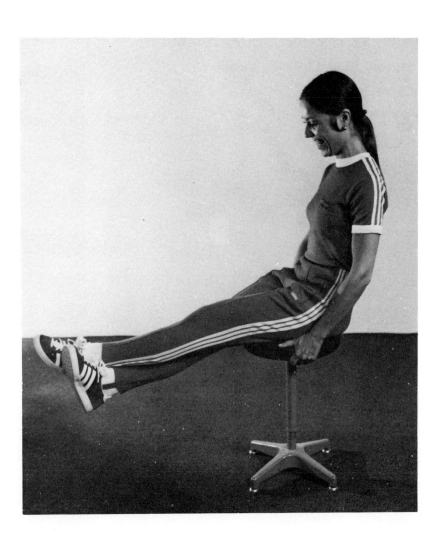

# EXERCISE 12   THREE-QUARTER SQUAT

## Purpose: Strengthen leg muscles

### Starting Position

Stand in doorway on a chair or low table. Place hands palms up on underside of top of door.

### Action

Holding three-quarter squat position, push up with legs.

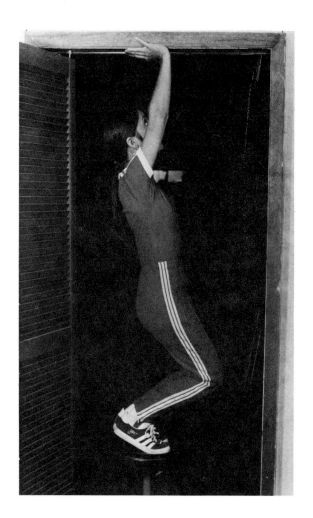

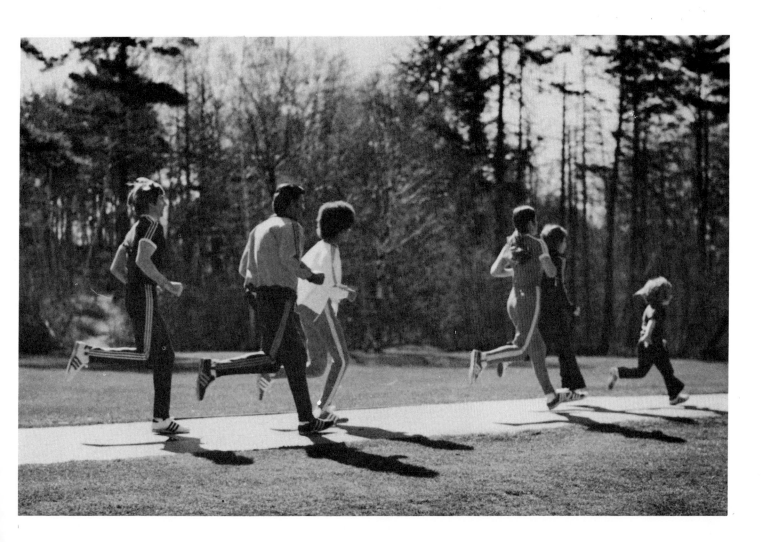

# A Strenuous But Reliable Motor Efficiency Test of Fitness

## FOR MEN AND WOMEN

The exercises in this test are designed to test seven significant aspects of fitness: Balance, Flexibility, Agility, Co-ordination, Strength, Power, and Endurance. If you can complete as specified 13 of the 20 exercises shown, you can consider yourself just barely fit.

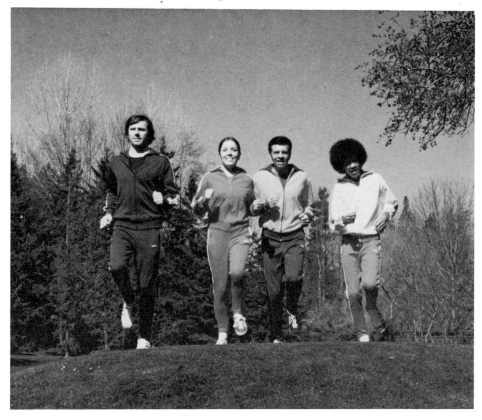

## BALANCE

### Exercise

1. Closed-Eyed Diver's Stance on Toes

### Action

Assume a diver's stance, arms outstretched, standing on toes with eyes closed. *Hold for 30 Seconds*

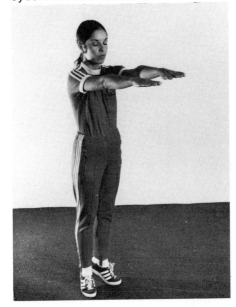

Pass ☐          Fail ☐

## 2. Squat Hand Stand

Squat with your palms on floor. Tip forward, resting legs on elbows, toes off the ground, head forward but not touching floor. *Hold for 15 Seconds*

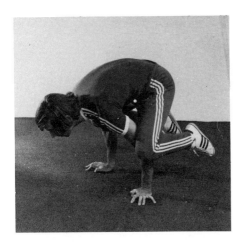

Pass ☐          Fail ☐

## 3. Circle Rotate

With your finger touching floor (left or right hand), walk in a circle around it 10 times in no more than 30 seconds. *Then walk a straight line for 10 feet within 5 seconds.*

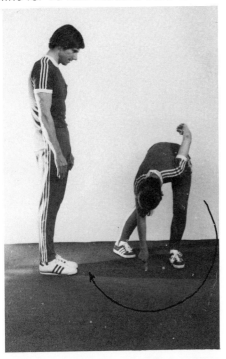

Pass ☐          Fail ☐

# FLEXIBILITY

## 4. Floor Touch

Keeping legs together and knees straight, bend at waist and touch floor with fingers. Women should touch floor with palms.

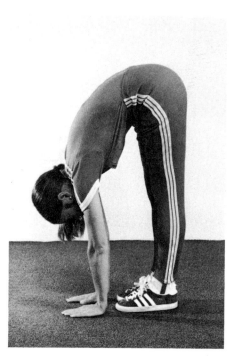

Pass ☐      Fail ☐

## 5. Trunk Flexion Forward

Slowly bend from sitting position, knees straight, until your forehead touches two fists, one atop the other on floor.

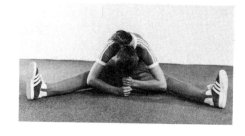

Pass ☐      Fail ☐

## 6. Trunk Extension Backward

Lying on stomach with feet pinned to floor and hands behind neck, raise chin up 18 inches from floor.

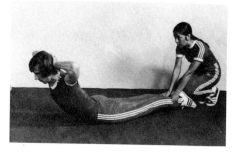

Pass ☐      Fail ☐

## AGILITY

### 7. Kneeling Jump

Kneel with insteps flat on the floor. Using just back and arms spring erect, both feet together. *Hold your balance for 3 seconds.*

### 8. Jack-Spring

From a standing position, jack-spring from the floor, touching toes at waist height. Bend legs only slightly. *Repeat 5 times in rapid succession.*

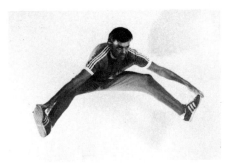

Pass ☐          Fail ☐

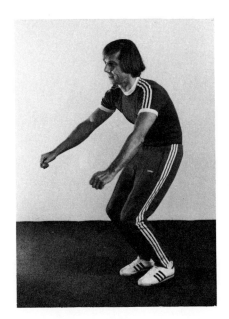

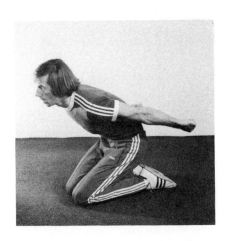

Pass ☐          Fail ☐

## 9. Six-Count Agility Sequence

In rapid succession perform the following 6 motions: 1. Squat, 2. Kick legs backward, 3. Kick legs forward through arms, 4. Turn over, 5. Squat, 6. Stand. *Repeat sequence 6 times in 30 Seconds.*

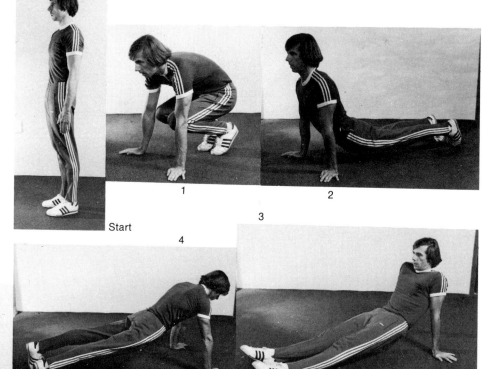

Start

1

2

3

4

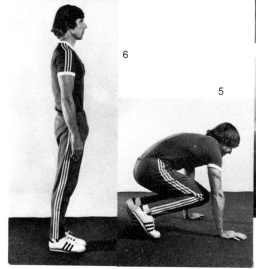

6

5

Pass ☐ Fail ☐

164

## CO-ORDINATION

10. Stride Jump with Variable Arm Raise

Simultaneously while stride jumping, arms are raised one to the side shoulder high and the other to the front and over head. With each stride jump, the position of arms is reversed. *Repeat sequence 10 times in rapid succession.*

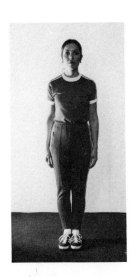
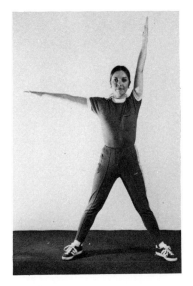
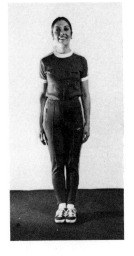
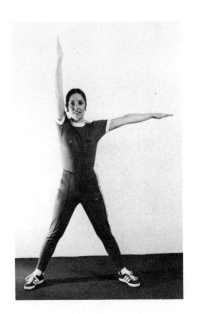

Pass ☐          Fail ☐

## 11. Double Stride Jump with Arm Raise

While doing a stride jump 2 counts out and 2 counts feet together, arms are raised over head and down to the sides on a 1–2 count. *Repeat full sequence 10 times in rapid succession.*

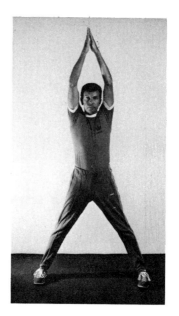

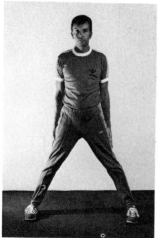

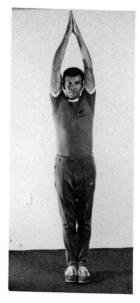

Pass ☐           Fail ☐

## STRENGTH

### 12. Body Lift

Lift and carry partner, fireman style (Partner within 10 pounds of your own weight) from his/her supine position face-up on floor. *Lift from floor to carry position in 10 seconds.*

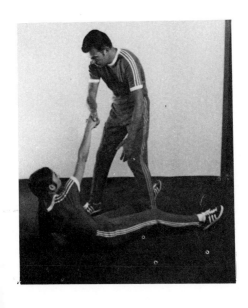

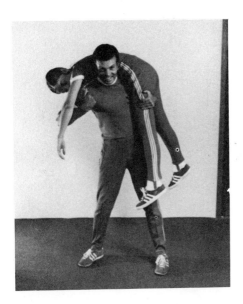

### 13. Rigid Body Hold

With arms at sides and back of head on partner's knee or edge of chair or bench, hold body rigid. *Hold for 30 seconds.*

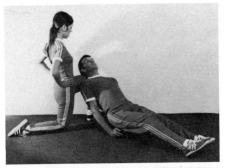

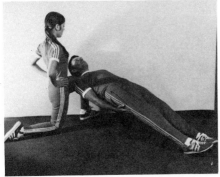

Pass ☐               Fail ☐     Pass ☐                    Fail ☐

### 14. Extended Push-Up

Lying on stomach, arms fully extended, lift body 6 inches off floor. Use just hands and toes. Women may use forearms. *Hold 15 seconds.*

Pass ☐　　　　　　Fail ☐

## POWER

### 15. Standing Broad Jump

Execute a standing broad jump the height you are plus 1 foot.

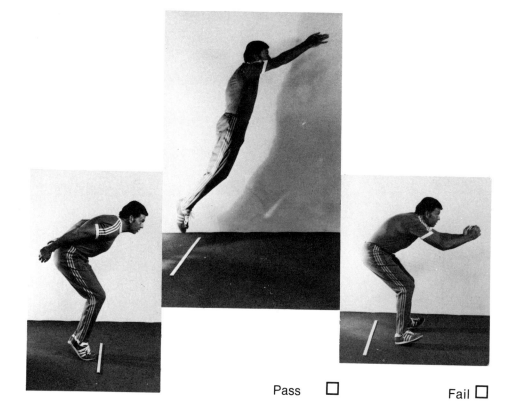

Pass ☐　　　　　　Fail ☐

## ENDURANCE

### 16. Full Push-Ups

Lying on floor position, hands beneath shoulders, execute 15 push-ups. Keep back straight. *Complete in 25 seconds.*

Pass ☐                    Fail ☐

### 17. Straddle Chinning

Lie on back, straddled by a partner, grasp partner's hands, and pull up until your elbows are at your sides. *Men repeat 20 times. Women repeat 10 times.*

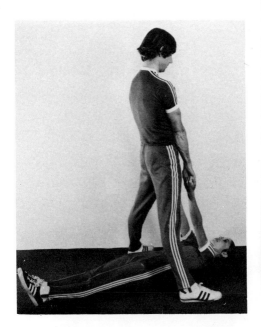
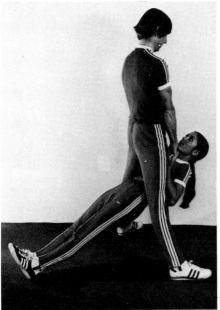

Pass ☐                    Fail ☐

## 18. V-Sit and Hold

Assume V-sit position with knees stiff and hands on hips or outstretched. DON'T FORGET TO BEND YOUR BACK. *Hold position for 60 seconds.*

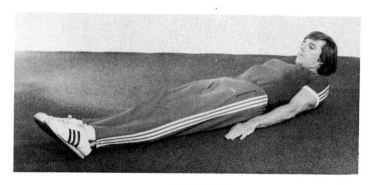

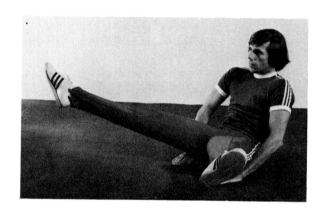

Pass ☐ Fail ☐

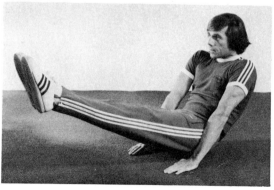

## 19. Breath Holding

Breathing normally, run on spot for 2 minutes at double time (180 steps per minute), then take three breaths. *Hold third breath for 30 seconds.*

Pass ☐ Fail ☐

## 20. Endurance Hops

Without stopping do:
1. 200 straddle hops
2. 200 scissor strides
3. 50 hops on left foot
4. 50 hops on right foot
5. 50 squat jumps.

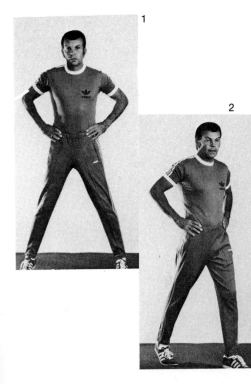

1

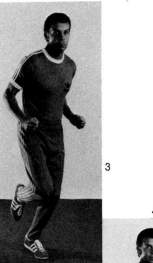

2

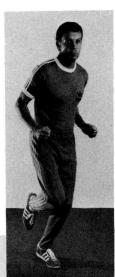

3

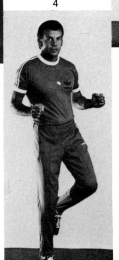

4

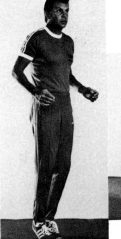

5-1

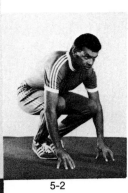

5-2

Pass ☐                    Fail ☐

Total Score: _____

**Note:** There are many variations of this test and I do not presume to suggest, therefore, that I have solely designed it. This particular version, however, is the adaptation I use and the number of repetitions and times suggested are the most widely accepted.

# Physical Fitness Quiz

Answer either True or False for each.

1. The average person reaches peak physical fitness at age 26.   T or F
2. Walking is not a sufficiently intense activity to help in improving cardiovascular (heart) fitness.   T or F
3. Sleep is the best remedy for chronic fatigue.   T or F
4. Children are equipped for sustained physical exercise.   T or F
5. Diet is the best method of losing weight.   T or F
6. It is advisable to continue exercising if you have a cold.   T or F
7. To be strong is to be fit.   T or F
8. Hardening of the arteries is a natural part of getting older.   T or F
9. Regular exercise increases one's resistance to most disease germs.   T or F
10. After a few years of normal office-type work, not one North American in 50 is physically fit.   T or F
11. A person can keep fit by exercising for less than one per cent of the week.   T or F
12. Regular exercise lengthens life.   T or F
13. Boredom can cause as much sickness as bacteria.   T or F
14. The human heart is a muscle.   T or F
15. Smoking fewer than 10 cigarettes per day has no effect on death rates.   T or F
16. Gaining weight is a natural effect of aging.   T or F
17. Improving one's cardiovascular (heart) fitness reduces the resting heart rate.   T or F
18. Getting winded means your lungs are not doing their work.   T or F
19. Height and weight tables are the best way to determine what you should weigh.   T or F
20. Athletic ability and co-ordination are important to the development of fitness.   T or F
21. Exercise can cause heart damage.   T or F
22. Exercising alone is just as good as exercising in a group.   T or F
23. After an intensive workout or a run it is a good idea to sit down and rest immediately.   T or F

24. Stretching exercises should only be done when the muscles are warmed up.     T or F
25. Exercises have to hurt if they are to be of sufficient intensity to provide significant benefits.     T or F
26. Regular exercise reduces blood pressure.     T or F

## Answers To Physical Fitness Quiz

1. TRUE. The age of 26 marks the average person's physical peak between the growing adolescent period and the levelling-off middle-age period.
2. FALSE. A brisk walk, if sustained for approximately 30 minutes, 4 times or more per week is sufficient to produce an improvement in cardiovascular (heart) fitness.
3. FALSE. Often, after a day of routine or frustration, a brisk workout or a walk will leave you refreshed and relieve fatigue.
4. TRUE. Exercise, no matter how strenuous, is not harmful to children, provided they are in a good state of health and nutrition. Their hearts are like powerful motors in small cars.
5. FALSE. Reducing weight is simply a matter of expending more calories through muscular activity than one consumes in food and drink. The difference between expenditure and consumption is drawn from fat stored in the body and this results in weight loss.
6. TRUE. Moderate exercise will improve your circulation, which in turn is the key to general fitness.
7. FALSE. Total physical fitness means a body developed in six areas: Strength, Balance, Power, Flexibility, Agility and Endurance.
8. FALSE. Hardening of the arteries can occur at any age. It is often the result of an inactive way of life. The best way to keep blood vessels open and prevent hardening of the arteries is through regular, rhythmic exercise.
9. FALSE. Bacteria are not fought with muscles or heart power. Resistance to germs is closely related to good nutrition and to specific antibodies found in blood and tissue.

10. TRUE. After a few years of normal office-type work, not one North American in fifty has even fairly good tone in the abdominal muscles.
11. TRUE. A good level of fitness can be maintained by 3 workouts of 30 minutes each week. This adds up to 1½ hours a week which is .89% of the 168 hours in a week.
12. FALSE. There is no good evidence that exercise either lengthens or shortens life. It does however help prevent premature aging and can lead you to a more alert and fuller life.
13. TRUE. The person with stomach trouble or throbbing headaches may be just plain bored. Finding new interests and exercising can help relieve such problems.
14. TRUE. The human heart is a muscle. Like all muscles it needs exercise and the right kind of exercise makes it grow stronger.
15. FALSE. Studies in Canada, Great Britain and the United States show that death rates for those who smoke less than 10 cigarettes per day are 40 per cent higher than for those who do not smoke.
16. FALSE. Ideally, an individual's weight should not exceed that which it was at age 25.
17. TRUE. A reduction of resting heart rate is one of the effects of improving the efficiency of the heart. Since it is able to pump more blood per beat, it need not beat as frequently. (A reduction in resting heart rate from 80 to 75 beats per minute saves 2,628,000 beats per year. At the rate of 75 beats per minute, this is equivalent to 24.33 DAYS of heart beats per *year*.)
18. FALSE. The "winded" feeling is a result of the heart's failure to keep up with the demands of the exercise. The lungs are involved to some extent, but the major factor is the efficiency of the heart muscle.
19. FALSE. Various muscle developments mean that two people with the same height may have quite different weights. The vital factor is how much of the weight is composed of excess fat.
20. FALSE. Some of the best activities for the development of fitness (walking, running, bicycling, etc) require very little skill or athletic talent.

21. FALSE. The normal healthy body has enough built-in safety devices to ensure that you can not hurt your heart by exercise. If, however, there is already heart damage, excessive exercise may irritate this situation or cause further damage. People of all ages with a known heart condition should first consult their doctor.
22. TRUE. The social environment is not the important factor; however, it sometimes encourages a greater degree of participation. What is important is that you enjoy what you are doing. An activity which is not enjoyed is generally not continued.
23. FALSE. It is essential that you cool down gradually to allow the blood to redistribute itself to all areas of the body. Failure to do this can cause lightheadedness and may even cause you to pass out due to a lack of oxygen being supplied to the brain.
24. TRUE. Cold muscles are most easily torn. Warm muscles are most easily stretched.
25. FALSE. If the exercise hurts you are probably doing too much too fast. You should exercise until you can feel the strain however.
26. FALSE. There is no conclusive proof that lower blood pressure is directly attributable to regular exercise. Exercise, however, does help in controlling weight and relieving stress, both of which are factors which affect blood pressure.